insatiable

insatiable

*a memoir
of love addiction*

Shary Hauer

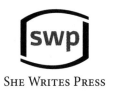

SHE WRITES PRESS

Published 2015
Printed in the United States of America
ISBN: 978-1-63152-982-5
Library of Congress Control Number: 2014957853

For information, address:
She Writes Press
1563 Solano Ave #546
Berkeley, CA 94707

She Writes Press is a division of SparkPoint Studio, LLC.

For my mother and father,
with deep love and enormous gratitude.

Confront the dark parts of yourself, and work to banish them with illumination and forgiveness. Your willingness to wrestle with your demons will cause your angels to sing.

August Wilson

Contents

Introduction

I had our entire future together mapped out before we had even met. For months, I had been reading in the morning newspaper about Robert, a prominent national consultant contracted by the city of St. Petersburg, Florida to help reduce its escalating homeless population. Robert wasn't a sit-behind-the-desk kind of consultant. He didn't shower for days, wore disguises, roamed the streets at night, and slept on grimy sidewalks to embed himself in the homeless community. I'd been volunteering for the homeless for twenty-plus years and had never heard of anyone at his level who lived among the homeless, Mother Teresa–style. A selfless servant. My kindred spirit. I had to meet this guy!

I e-mailed the city's homeless liaison to find out when Robert would next be presenting his findings to the City Council. "You just missed his presentation yesterday," she replied. He was returning to his home in Texas at the end of week, but she gave me his e-mail address. I sent an introductory note saying I'd love to glean some of his strategies to decrease homelessness over a cup of coffee the next time he was in town.

He responded right away: "Boy, it seems we have a lot in common. I'd love to get together." It was that easy. I was convinced the universe was pushing us together.

Less than forty-eight hours later, Robert and I were sipping cabernet and dining on steamed mussels and grouper in a popular bistro on Beach Drive in downtown St. Pete. I sat mesmerized by his stories of how he befriended his homeless brethren on the streets, was a White

1

House fellow, and how he'd served on a special diplomatic mission in Bahrain.

As he spoke, my long-held vision of traveling the globe with my beloved life partner and serving the world's hungry and homeless unfolded before me. At last I had met my match. I had found the man who fit the part I'd been auditioning for my entire life. An intelligent, gifted, deeply purposeful humanitarian whose soul's calling was dedicated to helping the most vulnerable. We set a date to meet for dinner on the beach the following month, when we'd both be back in town from our respective travels.

Immediately, I started reconfiguring my life around him. I had to get a bigger bed—he was six foot two—and a slew of new dresses and Botox. I'd needed to book hair and nail appointments. Get a bottle of Shalimar. And shimmery body butter. A lingerie overhaul was essential. The kitchen required a new coat of paint, and I had to call the landscaping guy. Then order new silk sheets and fluffy towels. I was manic, wired, not sleeping for days. The frenetic high of a cocaine-like craving. FOR CHRIST'S SAKE, WE HADN'T EVEN HAD A SECOND DATE!

In 2009, when I first discovered there was a name for my "affliction," I was floored. Yet deep down, I'd always known there was such a thing as love addiction. In fact, as far back as 1991, when I was in my first relationship after my divorce, I jokingly called myself a love addict. But when Patrick swooped in to rescue me and the floodgates of my obsessiveness burst, I had absolutely no clue that love addiction was a serious, sometimes fatal, psychological disorder—potentially as lethal as heroin or alcohol addiction.

The tricky part about love addiction, unlike alcohol, drug, and other addictions, is that people don't take it seriously. They don't think of it as a bona fide addiction. I didn't. Plus, being lovesick is glorified. You're supposed to feel giddy and crazy when you're in love, right?

Up until a few years ago, I had no earthly idea that relationships were my drug.

I did not realize that the excitement—the uncertainty, the torment, the "Does he want me?," "Will he call me?," "Why didn't he call me?,"

"When is he coming back?"—was not love. I'd always associated the intensity and drama of my rocky relationships with real intimacy. Why else, then, would I be bored to tears with the good guys—the kind, secure, reliable men who adored me? What's more, I was so gullible—so starved for attention and love that I'd distort the significance of a man's slightest compliment. I'd take wild leaps to certainty. Worse, I got sucked in by men who supersized their attention and poured it on fast and furious. Although I initially doubted their intentions, it didn't stop me from gobbling up their innuendos and digging my claws into them, as if they were my last meal, convinced each one was "*the* one."

I am a love addict. I am a relationship addict. A romance addict. According to Love Addicts Anonymous (LAA), there are several types of love addicts. And many, like me, have multiple, overlapping, sometimes contradictory addictions: codependent love addiction, obsessive love addiction, romance addiction, relationship addiction, and so on.

My high was the anticipation, the fantasy, the romance, the rush of a new relationship. I got into and stayed in relationships not because I fell in love with the man but because I craved being wanted. I needed a man in order to be more of a woman. When I wasn't in a relationship, I felt dead. I perked up, resuscitated, looked better, talked better, and felt better when there was promise of a new relationship. The anticipation of fresh love. A fresh source of adoration. It was never really about the man. Rather, it was the romance, being the object of someone's desire. That's what gave me a surge, a rush. Made me feel powerful. The man was secondary.

I was what most therapists would call a high-functioning love addict. I woke up every morning passionate, enthusiastic, and purposeful. I hit the gym. I had many friends and a successful corporate career. I founded a firm where I coached high-powered executives. People saw me as in charge, superconfident, and independent. But at night, behind closed doors, I lived a double life—secretly and unconsciously deflating all my power, wanting nothing more than to be magically rescued and taken care of by my majestic king.

In most of my relationships, I was the fixer, the savior, especially with men who were needy in some way. The eldest of six children, lacking the nurturing and love I needed, I became the caregiver, the little mother from age two. When it came to chasing love by refurbishing men, no job was beneath me. I served as career advisor, chef, chief motivational officer, mother, dog sitter, dance instructor, drill sergeant, baker, résumé writer, travel agent, image consultant, minister, therapist, chauffeur, doctor, nurse, and bank. Anything to win and keep the man who would love, cherish, and protect me the rest of my days. It would take many years before I realized my pattern of feeling utterly worthless without a man by my side.

Like an alcoholic who drinks to black out, I overdosed on too many wrong relationships. Trying too hard to be loved, I overfixed, overcaretook, overmothered, overstepped. I got in and overstayed in relationships to eke out some semblance of love, attempting in desperate ways to quiet my carnivorous longing to be tended to and cherished. But I knew only the fleeting, unpredictable kind of love—the kind of love that abandoned, caused pain. And although it took me months, sometimes years, to recover from a breakup, I always ended up with the same self-loathing and remorse that alcoholics speak of: "Why did I do it? I knew better." But it was all I knew.

In comparison to the horror stories of many addicts—those raised by drunken, drug-addicted mothers who abandoned their children at age three; those repeatedly sexually abused by fathers; or those who endured worse—my upbringing was tame. I was raised by good and decent parents. It's only in recent years that I've begun to understand that I was a highly sensitive and insecure person who had been emotionally neglected as a child. Endlessly searching for a sign that I was appreciated, valued, and loved, I came up empty. When I was five, I unknowingly created a fantasy life of being rescued by the classic fairy-tale knight in shining armor. That fantasy remained imbedded and played out in episode after episode in my twenties, thirties, forties, and even fifties.

The past nearly twenty-five years of my life have been an excruciating odyssey, one man at a time. From the bottom of despair, clinical depression, and hopelessness—through decades of cravings, highs, fixes, and withdrawals to abstinence, understanding, and acceptance—I am relearning how to love myself rather than depending on a man to do it for me.

My savior and constant companion on this long, hellish trek was my journal. For more than two decades, it was the place I went to celebrate, rant, agonize, and mourn every exhilarating new relationship and devastating breakup. It's where I prayed and pleaded and processed a mountain of books and web sites in hopes of understanding why my love life was littered with failure. There were no epiphanies, just a steady, potholed, ever-hopeful march that led to me to stumble upon something called love addiction. Finally I had found a name and an explanation for the self-destructive pattern I was chained to. Perhaps you are stuck in your own version of love hell. By sharing my experiences and the lessons I've learned along the way, my deepest hope is that you, too, will begin to free yourself and find peace with or without a partner.

1
Under a Spell

Up until 1983, my life had been pretty predictable. At twenty-six, I'd never been in trouble at home or with the law, unless you count the time I was slapped by Sister Rose Marie in the eighth grade. I'd never been impetuous as a teenager—not like my brother Mike, who seemed to run away from home every week. And rarely was I spontaneous. I was the classic Catholic "good girl" from the get-go. God-fearing and mom-petrified, I was a guardian of right and wrong, constantly keeping watch over my five younger siblings for missteps. I guess that's how I ended up doing the same as manager of strategic promotions for a 53,000-employee international company headquartered in Dayton, Ohio: mother-henning, making sure my team behaved professionally, and was well thought of by the higher-ups.

And there I was that Saturday night, walking into our division's Christmas party, a potential cesspool of bacchanalia. My date, Bob—a casual friend I occasionally went out with—and I tiptoed from the icy parking lot, shook the snowflakes off our coats, and strolled through the massive oak front door into NCR Country Club's decked-out salon. The Christmas party was always a grand affair, with dinner and dancing for the nearly three hundred employees of Product Marketing and their dates.

I usually dreaded those parties. The obligatory small talk with spouses, awkward conversation with senior management, and endless appreciative smiles required so much energy. But that year I felt especially festive. It was the first time I was with a date. Thank God

I wouldn't have to endure the night alone, feigning confidence but secretly bereft without a man by my side. I couldn't stand to be alone.

Bob was preppy handsome, tall with sandy hair and an intellectual air. He was also a little reserved, likely a prerequisite for being a manager in the staid Accounting Department. We'd met on the company softball team in the spring, something my coworker and friend Kate had encouraged me to join, despite my protests.

"You'll have a blast. And look at the new people you'll meet. You never know. Go have some fun instead of working so much." She was right. I worked late every night, and despite endlessly ruminating about men and dating, I hadn't had a date with any potential, much less a relationship, in an abysmal four years. I felt absolutely inadequate. But softball season was over and everything was different now. John had burst into my life. He was a colleague in Product Marketing, and we started working together on a project. He was in a five-year marriage. And we were having an affair. It was brand new; we'd been seeing each other for less than two months—discreetly, of course. But already he was my all. He'd been coming over to my apartment after work a couple of nights during the week. Now, walking into the party, I was guarded. John was going to show up with his wife. I was with Bob. I had to keep it together. No one could know our secret.

Bob guided me to the bar for a glass of Chablis. In the alcove to our right, couples stood in line to pose for a keepsake photo in front of a snowcapped alpine backdrop. I scanned the room looking for John. Across the vast living room, a twelve-foot Douglas fir glowed with what seemed like thousands of miniature white lights and old-fashioned gold glass balls. I couldn't help feel the holiday spirit. The place was gorgeous.

Wine glasses in hand, Bob and I wandered through the rooms, praising the gold-velvet-ribboned fresh pine wreaths adorning every nook. The succulent aroma of just-out-of-the-oven standing rib roast beckoned us to the buffet line, where dozens had gathered. *Why hadn't he called?* John had promised he'd call that afternoon. I needed to hear from him. To be reassured by him. I wanted to hear him say, "She means nothing to me anymore. It's over between us. Yes, she will be with me. Technically, we're still married. But you will be the only one on my mind tonight." I needed him to say these things. I waited by the phone all day, shoving aside going to the supermarket, the dry cleaners, and the hardware store to hear him say that. He'd be home from basketball by 12:30, he'd said. Maybe he had second thoughts about me. Maybe he had been with his wife all day and couldn't get away. Maybe I had misread his intentions when he had fixed his eyes on me with such intensity and love just three nights before. Maybe he didn't mean it when he blurted out, "I want to be with you forever." Maybe the last two months had meant nothing to him. And everything to me. I was bombarded with torturous self-doubt.

As Bob and I migrated to the buffet line, I heard laughter pealing from the enclosed patio behind us, where the DJ, dance floor, and more dining tables were set up. We turned to see a motley band of six men from the Retail Group arm in arm, lip-syncing "Grandma Got Run Over by a Reindeer." Mike, one of the group's managers and clearly the ringleader, waved at us, oblivious to the fact that he was spilling his beer down the side of his suit jacket. It was only 7:30, but the partying was well under way. It had been a grueling year for our hard-driving division—too many months of working early mornings and late nights. I could feel the tension and stress lift. Everyone was ready to make merry.

Still, it was a company party. I knew the rules. As a manager, I was cognizant of keeping the proper balance between festive and business. I'd never dream of letting loose, especially at a work function. It boggled my mind how others could allow themselves to lose control. Every year someone misbehaved, always under the judgmental eyes of senior management.

One year Andy, a closeted gay college intern in my department, typically reserved, apparently decided to come out at the Christmas party. With his dress shirt unbuttoned, gyrating his hips to the music and swinging his tie overhead, he did a holiday striptease in front of the vice president and a gathering crowd. Before I could inch in to stop Andy, the song ended. I knew I'd get the question Monday morning: "Who is this guy, and why did you hire him?" The year before that, Beth, a beloved member of my department with a loud barroom laugh, had too many Budweisers and entertained us in the ladies' room, mimicking the fake southern accent of our boss's wife, who just happened to be holed up in the last stall.

This year, I was determined to avoid another fiasco.

Then, out of the corner of my eye, I saw John poised near the dance floor, an attractive librarian-ish blond by his side. *Must be Betty*, I thought. *His wife.* He was cutting up, surrounded by four of his teammates and their dates. John was gregarious, a natural leader, six foot three with a booming presenter's voice. People paid attention when he was in the room.

"Is that Donna and her husband?" Bob motioned to the couple standing at the hors d'oeuvres table. I waved and mouthed, "Come join us." *Did he see me?*

The table was getting crowded and noisy with banter and laughs. My team loved working and socializing with one another. But tonight I was somewhere else, flooded by conflicting desires: I wanted to flee, run far away from this place. Now. Yet I needed to see him, be with him.

"Hi everybody," Donna said as she approached the table. "You all remember my husband, Rob, don't you?"

"Hi Rob," we all chimed.

Between bites, I took a quick gaze around the room again. John was in the same spot, looking at me, his penetrating blue eyes not blinking. *How long had he been watching me?* I wondered. A subtle smile creased his mustached lip. He winked. *Oh my God.* My stomach lurched in excitement. I turned back to my plate and the table conversation, taking a big gulp of water, trying to collect myself.

Seconds later, I put my fork down. I stood up and walked away. From Bob. And all the others. Without a word. No "I'm getting some more salad. Would anyone like anything?" No "Excuse me, I'm going to the ladies' room." Nothing. I was silent. I wasn't thinking. I was only responding. Like a moth magnetized to the brightest light in the room, I was operating on instinct only: I need to be with him. I need to go to him now.

As if on cue, John walked toward me, reached for my hand, and escorted me to the dance floor. I loved the way he took charge, confident and commanding at twenty-six. He was so debonair and sexy in his three-piece charcoal gray suit and cherry-red silk tie. He drew me in, his determined hands holding tight to my waist, and whispered in my ear,

"You are so beautiful."

God, how I loved hearing those words from him, even though I struggled to believe them.

"Thank you," I murmured. *Did he mean it? Really mean it?* I hungered for his attention, any attention. I craved being desired.

How could he know that I had spent nearly the entire day getting ready for the party? Getting ready for him? How could he know that I had taken my new black velvet dress out of the closet and its plastic bag at eight that morning, inspected it, and methodically brushed any lint away in long up-and-down strokes? That I had soaked in an hour-long bubble bath spiked with luxurious bath oil beads, shaving my legs twice? That I had double-checked my perfectly manicured nails at least four times, envisioning his hands, his body covering mine? That my red bra and panties were freshly spritzed with Shalimar?

A hint of his Halston cologne rested in my nose. My body relaxed in the familiarity of him. *I'm safe. I'm home.* It had been three unbearable days since I had been in his arms. I'd been unable to think about anything else. Other than him. And us. And the next time.

In the background, Lionel Richie's soulful voice implored us to explore our love. John and I moved in tandem, our eyes glued on each other. His wife, Betty, watched expressionless from the sidelines. My date, Bob, sat alone across the room.

Why wasn't I overwhelmed with paranoia about what people were thinking? Why wasn't I insane with worry about how Betty was feeling? How could I have been so cold and dismissive of Bob? How could I have violated my own sacrosanct "Christmas party rules"? Why wasn't I concerned about the consequences? How could I, the obedient "good girl" who had never been in one iota of trouble, find herself on the dance floor, seductively shaking her hips in the arms of a married man at a company party? What could I have been thinking?

The short answer: I wasn't.

It's difficult for me to understand how I could have been that unconscious. But I realize now that I was under a spell. Absolutely and totally fixated with a desperate desire to be loved.

"You are the sun, you are the rain . . . you need to know, I love you so," Lionel sang. I was powerless. Hypnotized. This successful, popular, handsome man wanted me. Me! I was drunk with the possibility of us. For once in my life, I was oblivious to who was watching. What they were thinking. Consequences. None of that mattered.

From the beginning, the relationship was fraught with allure and tension. I'd noticed a shift in John within a week or two of our departments' starting to work together on a significant new computer product launch. He visited my cubicle more frequently, inventing lame business reasons to stop by. He stayed longer than usual. He looked at me with what seemed like desire. But he was married. I knew that. He was off-limits.

"No, no," he said at a "working" lunch a week later. "I'm separated. We're getting a divorce. It's in the works now." Soon we were sneaking away from the office, signing out to go to a photo shoot at the product studio or a meeting at the brochure printer. Instead we'd rendezvous at a nearby warehouse, where I'd park my car and slide into his silver Porsche 924 and we'd grab each other, panting and necking like teenagers. I was lured by his confidence. I'd never been with anyone so self-assured. He was an up-and-coming leader and so was I. He knew what he wanted and how to get it. I didn't argue. I didn't get to vote. Only with my lips and welcoming bed. Yes, I was a walking contradiction. Here I was, a successful corporate woman who, by all appearances, had it *so* together. But, in matters of the heart, I assumed a new identity, shrinking into a subservient and dependent role. With John, I was in a trance, literally acting out my ultimate dream of being rescued by a majestic king for a lifetime of magical romance and sweet security. My dream was not a little girl's passing fantasy. It was my internal reality, a truth lodged deep inside my love-starved heart. It fueled me. Gave me purpose.

Less than three months into our affair, he stated his love, courting me fervently. Over Christmas break, while he was with his family in Virginia, he sent two dozen red roses, a golden ballotin of Godiva chocolates, and a flowery card expressing how he wished he could be with me on Christmas day. Grand romantic gestures were my most prized catnip, and with each orchestration, John ensnared me further.

After work, he would go to a meeting, play basketball in his Tuesday league, or perhaps go home to say hello and have dinner with his wife.

I never knew. I never asked. I trusted him. He was separated, getting a divorce. That's all I needed to know.

Some nights he'd come over to my third-floor one-bedroom apartment in a quiet tree-lined redbrick complex three miles from the office. Candles lit, the kitchen aromatic, my bedroom dimmed, and me perfumed and waiting. I lived in anticipation of our upcoming "dates"—imagining and reimagining the romantic possibilities. I was the stage director, envisioning and executing alluring scenes. Every prop—crystal goblets of cabernet, perfumed candlelight, his favorite dinner on the stove, Barry White's "Never, Never Gonna Give You Up" growling from the cassette deck—and every scene—the welcome-home kiss at the airport, a long walk under the harvest moon—was choreographed in my mind's eye. After midnight, he'd reach for the door and we'd still be standing on the stairwell kissing passionately an hour later. I couldn't let go, so hungry, so starving for his vigorous and certain love.

In April 1984, four months after the Christmas party and less than thirty days after his divorce was finalized, John and I got engaged. We celebrated at one of my favorite places—the historic Golden Lamb Inn in Lebanon, Ohio. It wasn't a surprise engagement—we had picked out the ring three weeks before—and he didn't get down on his knee to ask me for my hand. But when he opened the door to our room and I saw a dozen huge long-stemmed roses, a bottle of chilled champagne, and a blue-enveloped card awaiting, I gasped. I whirled around and smothered him with a long kiss.

"The last six months have been the most exciting time of my life," his card said. "You stir up emotions and feelings in me I never knew existed. I love you and want to spend the rest of my life with you. I love you, will you marry me? You will make me the happiest and proudest person on the face of this earth! Love always, John."

He reached for my hand. I looked into his eyes with the most conviction I've ever had about anything and said, "Yes. Of course I will."

Before dinner, after a glass or two of champagne, we goofed off, memorializing the occasion by taking photos of each other on the antique cherrywood double bed. The camera shook in my hands as

I laughed uncontrollably shooting John naked. He was beaming, his parts covered with a pillow, holding the bottle of champagne and a glass. In another photo, I lay in repose, my eyes shut. Wearing a plum wraparound dress, I solemnly held the vase of roses on my belly in a funereal pose, a smirk ready to burst.

We made love several times that night. Unable to sleep, I was giddy in love, juiced on romance and the thrill of us. This man—this strong, charming, exciting man—loved me, wanted me, intended to marry me!

All of it was a proverbial whirlwind, and before long it became more like a fierce tornado, speeding far too fast. And I was trapped in his vortex.

He wanted to get married right away—in July. "What better time to marry than in your birthday month?" he had said. I was touched. Surely, his impatience stemmed from his uncontrollable desire to be with me for the rest of his life. I couldn't stop the racing train, and I didn't want to. Yet I was overwhelmed and stressed. Working sixty hours a week, traveling—there was no way I could pull off a big wedding in three months. Plus, churches and reception venues were booked a year in advance. We agreed on September.

In every nonworking moment I was consumed with the details of planning a wedding and reception for nearly two hundred people, a process I thought I could manage with ease. Instead it turned into a stream of turmoil and tears.

During those few months, I didn't pause. I was unable to interpret John's lack of involvement in planning our wedding as anything more than "he's too busy." I never bothered to understand what had really happened in his marriage to Betty or what impact that might one day have on our relationship.

"We were just friends, just roommates," he said. "She didn't like big parties and roller coasters. And she liked to read." Somehow, that made sense to me back then. I didn't probe.

One night, two months before our wedding, I asked John, "What happens when we have a big disagreement or encounter difficulties?"

Without hesitating he said, "We'll get a divorce," as if divorce were as routine as replacing a flat tire. I didn't respond. Everything he said I accepted, but at some remote level I was troubled by his nonchalance.

I ignored the quiet voice whispering, *What in the hell are you doing?* John was more than I had hoped for. This was true love.

We were married on a rainy and chilly Saturday afternoon in late September.

The church was stunning. It had a classic neo-Gothic sanctuary, with soaring buttresses and hundreds of glowing candles. White tulle and hand-cut white lilies adorned each pew. Mammoth white floral arrangements blanketed the altar. The endless aisle was carpeted in white silk runners. At 4:00 p.m., the seven-thousand-pipe organ announced my arrival, Westminster chimes and the "Wedding March" processional booming majestically from the balcony. Arm in arm with my tuxedoed dad, I inched down the aisle in an elegant beaded and lace ivory gown. A gorgeous white bouquet, identical to Princess Di's, cascaded to the floor. It was all very regal. Exactly what I had dreamed.

Only our wedding was in a Presbyterian church in downtown Dayton, because my family parish—and every other Catholic parish— would not allow me to marry a divorced man. My father could not accept that ruling. He was certain his friendships with priests throughout the state, not to mention the tens of thousands of dollars he and his parents had stuffed into Sunday collection baskets over decades, would convince them otherwise. Unfortunately, it could not be done without an annulment, which would take a year or several.

Not one of my sisters but my best friend, Kathy, served as my maid of honor, which prompted one of many screaming matches with my mother. And the fact that John did not pick any of my brothers as ushers was the source of another tirade. Nothing I did seemed to go right. And to top it off, we were married by a female minister—a rarity in 1984 and an impossibility in the Catholic Church. I feared disappointing my grandparents. I had already done so with my parents. I was frazzled.

Our reception was a blur. I wasn't drunk, not even close. Yet I recall very little. Other than it was a grand affair our 150 or so guests and my bar-dancing brother, Mike, seemed to enjoy very much. We got back to our hotel room at midnight, and I was already dreading the

5:00 a.m. wakeup call to make our flight to Cancun. I cried myself to sleep that night. It's not exactly how I expected to feel on my first night of wedded bliss. Was it a release of all that pressure leading up to the wedding? Reality setting in? I didn't connect with my emotions back then. I was unable to discern why I was overwhelmed or to know what I was really feeling.

Once we returned from our honeymoon, I got right down to the business of being a devoted wife. I moved into John's simple 1960s ranch home, which he had shared with Betty. Although I was uncomfortable living in *their* place, it didn't occur to me to lobby for a new home that would be *our* home. John had declared, "This is where we're going to live." And I agreed.

As energetic, confident, and driven as I was in my career, at home I was passive. John drove the bus and made the decisions. And, apparently, I was happy to comply. I was determined to be the person I thought he wanted me to be. If I worked hard to show him my love, I was certain I'd earn and secure his lasting love. I'd do anything to please him, cooking his favorites like chicken-fried steak and chocolate oatmeal no-bake cookies. I shopped for new suits and ties to spruce up his professional image. I managed the household, the cleaning, the repairs and renovations. And, boy, did I have my hands full in that department. The decor was hideous. Gold-and-black wallpaper in the front entrance. Paper-thin indoor/outdoor patterned green-and-black carpet. Redbrick walls, wrought-iron gates, and an Italian gondola mural—all in the family room. Room by room, I had memories stripped and replaced. I did as much as I could without offending—which I ended up doing anyway. We almost came to blows when I wanted to move his favorite piece of art—a huge painting of a shipyard scene in garish oils—from the family room's central wall to the spare bedroom. He put his foot down when I begged him to let me replace the overstuffed, rust-colored velour couch and chair. "It's staying. That's final," he said.

John was gung ho to have children straight away. But I was twenty-seven and intent on moving up the corporate ladder. I didn't plan to have children until I was thirty. Naturally, he attempted to sell me on the idea, waving the most adorable pair of beaded suede infant moccasins he had bought on an Indian reservation years before.

"Won't our little boy look so cute in these?" he asked. Despite my mission to please him, baby-making was the one area in which I wasn't yet willing to negotiate.

· ·

The second October of our marriage, we went to homecoming weekend at John's alma mater, the University of Nebraska in Lincoln—home of the legendary Cornhusker team, zealous fans, and a stadium heralded as the "Cathedral of College Football." I couldn't wait to visit a state that seemed so wholesome and gosh-golly and teeming with good-natured farmers. The night before the homecoming game, fifty or so of his fellow 1979 classmates met at an off-campus pizza haunt for kegs of beer and pepperoni pies. *This will be fun,* I told myself. *I'm sure I'll love all his friends.* But as soon as we walked in, John raced across the room to surprise attack his former roommate, and he was off in his own world the rest of the night. He chatted, joked, and flirted, and he neglected to introduce me, much less check on me to see if I needed another drink. Self-conscious and socially shy, I didn't have the confidence back then to simply go up and meet people on my own. Instead I sat on a stool in the corner alone, occasionally smiling, pretending to be having a good time watching my husband ignore me for three hours. I noticed all the other couples together, laughing, hugging, reveling in one another's company. *Is John embarrassed by me? Why did he bring me?* I wondered. Rather than be concerned about his behavior, I chalked his disregard up to his extreme extroversion, one of his gifts that I was in awe of.

My main wifely duty was to serve as John's number-one cheerleader. I listened to his work stories, which dominated most of our alone time. I encouraged and stroked him endlessly. His career and reputation were paramount, his ambition to advance heavy-duty.

Many years later, when I read greeting cards John had given me for my birthday and Valentine's Day in the first two years of our marriage, it was clear what drew him to me. "With you by my side, there will be no limit to my success," he wrote. "You are my guiding light to happiness and success," read another. Success. I was to be his ticket

to success. True enough. I was a good corporate wife, an asset. I was
well liked by my coworkers, highly regarded by the senior management team. When John and I first met, my black BMW 318i was just
a few months old. Looking back, I'm sure his mouth secretly watered
when he saw my car. My manager's salary combined with his director's salary could make for a sizable increase. A bigger this, a bigger
that. And that's exactly what happened. Except a bigger family. After
our first year of marriage, John did a complete 360 on having babies.
All of a sudden, he announced, "I'm selfish. I want time for sports
and work." But I wasn't concerned. I knew I'd be able to convince him
otherwise when I was ready.

We stayed in our ranch for nearly two years before we decided to
buy a new home. I was ready for a place that could be ours, perhaps
a 1930s Tudor with creaky polished oak floors, hidden alcoves, and
soaring evergreens. John wanted a new and larger house, a trophy to
display his burgeoning professional status. Although I thought I had
made a convincing pitch, I was overruled. Once he saw the modern
two-story, all-brown box with four bedrooms, baby-blue carpet,
a deck and pool in the backyard, a recreation room with a billiards
table, and—the pièce de résistance—a basketball hoop in the driveway, it was a done deal. John's party house. He could hardly contain
himself. It wasn't worth making a big fuss over. Again, I went along. I
loved him. I was dedicated to his happiness, to the cause of us.

Our first summer in the house, we had a barbecue for forty of our
coworkers on a sweltering July Saturday afternoon. I greeted everyone at the front door, prepared all the food, grilled the hamburgers,
directed people to the bathrooms, grabbed more towels, sweated
bullets in the ninety-degree heat, and scowled. Where was John?
Whooping it up in the pool volleyball game, oblivious to me running
around, up to my eyeballs in hamburger grease. I wanted him to be
happy, to have fun. If I was upset at his lack of help, I rarely expressed
it. Sacrifice—that's what I thought married people did. I'd do anything
to keep him happy and to keep us together.

When John got promoted to vice president to head up an important
new software group for the company in Columbia, South Carolina,
the powers that be created a manager of product promotions position
for me at the sister plant about five hundred feet across the street from

John's facility. I was so proud of him. We were excited about a new start.

In November 1988 we bought a charming Charleston-style row house with a mother-in-law suite on Lake Murray, literally in the sticks in Chapin, forty minutes from the office. I loved the idea of living on the water, a quiet refuge with one or two neighbors who were camouflaged by sturdy stands of white pine. Only months later did I realize that there was just one restaurant, Lizard's Thicket, two miles away and that the library, a fifteen-mile jaunt, was the size of a closet and had uninteresting books. I figured most of what I needed would be close by, but it turned out there was no gym, no bookstore, no nothing but lakefront. And that's exactly what appealed to John. He wanted a speedboat in the worst way, envisioning rousing barbecue weekends, this time with a party boat for waterskiing and inner-tubing.

John did buy a boat. But he was absorbed in his new job, traveling every week, hiring dozens of specialists from all over the world, building an organization from scratch. He was rarely home. And I was a proverbial fish out of water in my new position. I worked alongside eight hundred engineers. Mostly men. All white. Largely native South Carolinians. Technical, dry, quiet. I had spent my entire career working with vibrant, fun sales and marketing people from all over the world. What was I going to do? I was isolated at work and at home. No friends. No social life. Empty.

I felt abandoned. When John was home, I scrounged for a compliment, a hug, a promise of some alone time over the upcoming weekend. He was my sun. I orbited around him. I thought you were supposed to orbit each other when you were married. Back then, I was oblivious to a lot of things: (1) I didn't see how I had idealized John, put him on a pedestal, begun to view him as superior to me in many ways. I didn't see that I had attached myself to his identity. (2) I didn't see that I hadn't cultivated my own life. How I had abandoned my own interests over the previous four years. How I had sacrificed and invested all of me in him. How I was the constant caretaker and pleaser. (3) I didn't see that he wasn't romantic anymore. I poured it on him constantly, complimenting him, but he rarely expressed his ardor.

Rather, he teased me. When he was asked why he had married me, he'd love to tell people, "It was her high arches." I had very high arches and couldn't wear normal pumps or sling-back shoes. They didn't fit; my instep towered over the side of the shoe. So I had to find shoes with an opening on the inside, a cutout. John called them blowouts.

He saw me sitting on the bed every morning, struggling to squeeze into my requisite corporate panty hose. "Are you having trouble again with your sausage casings?" he'd shout from the bathroom.

And when I happened to be side by side with him in the bathroom, putting on my makeup, he'd remark in a disgusted tone, "God, you're sure putting on a lot of spackle this morning."

Of course, it was funny. We always laughed. I couldn't acknowledge that I was hurting.

Despite it all, I was convinced this was the perfect time to start a family. I was now thirty-one and was ready to have a baby. My new job was less demanding. I finally had room in my life to focus on creating our family.

On one of John's rare nights in town, he invited me to have dinner with Lew, the senior vice president's chief of staff, at a restaurant in downtown Columbia. Lew was in town from headquarters for a few days of meetings with John's new team. I loved Lew. I had worked with him in Dayton on a backbreaking yearlong special project. He was one of the most gracious, polished, and thoughtful leaders in the company.

"So, when are you two going to start having kids?" he asked, sipping his scotch and soda.

I looked at John, hoping he'd respond. But he was silent, disengaged.

"I know. It's about time, isn't it?" I said. "John's been gone so much. It's been tough to find the time to talk."

"Just put a business plan together and we'll discuss it," John said. He forked another slab of steak, impatient to get to the next item on his agenda.

A stab of rejection clenched my gut. *Maybe he's joking. He was trying to be funny, right?* No. He was not laughing.

I managed to look up at Lew, who seemed as surprised and uncomfortable as I was.

By this point, other women would have said, "I'm done. I'm not going to do this anymore." For me, that line of thinking was as remote as the Antarctic. I had not one iota of doubt about us. I was hooked. Nothing was more essential to me than winning and keeping John's love. No matter how many times I had to win it. His occasional mean jabs? I had a high tolerance for pain. Loneliness? I was accustomed to feeling isolated. Lack of emotional connection? I had a lot of experience in that department.

I'd simply try harder. There had to be something I hadn't figured out yet. Hadn't done enough of yet. I would be more loving. I would find new ways to please him, to be more helpful, to lessen his stress. I would give all that I had to this man, the man I believed was fully capable of giving me the love and attention I needed.

2
The Good Girl

Two weeks after their honeymoon in Acapulco in October 1956, my mother and father drove cross-country from Dayton, Ohio, to Santa Ana, California, so my father could begin his assignment as a second lieutenant in the US Marine Corps. They settled into a two-bedroom, gray, slab rental home on the El Toro Marine Corps Air Station, tucked within a hundred-thousand-acre ranch of ambrosial orange groves and strawberry fields. The plan was for my mother to get a job as a secretary, ideally on the base, and to work for a few years before they returned to Ohio to start a family.

But three weeks later, after dragging around with no energy, feeling dizzy and light-headed and believing her body was rebelling against Southern California's climate, my mom went to the doctor, fearful something was desperately wrong. Instead she was shocked to learn that she was pregnant with me. Sick for weeks, she was in no position to start a new job. Instead, she settled in and accepted her new unfamiliar life course as housewife and mother.

Will I be a good mother? Do I even want to be a mother? I imagine my mother asking herself these questions during those wildly hormonal months. If my mother, at twenty-five, was a reluctant mother, I certainly couldn't blame her.

My mother was unmothered and unfathered. She was the child of a one-night stand. A one-afternoon stand is more the truth, actually. She was born in Appalachian Ohio to an eighteen-year-old mother who had had sex with a neighbor boy who slipped into her family's cabin on a bleak January day. That boy moved away soon after and was never in my mother's life. It didn't get much better after that.

One frigid winter night when my mother was three, dusk turning to black, a foot of snow on the ground, Clara, my mother's mother, was anxious to get to the Virginia Inn for a night of flirting, dancing, and boozing. Walking from their little, white-frame house, Clara grabbed my mother's hand, pulling her impatiently along the hills of desolate Gee Hollow, a mile away. Who knows where her husband, Cisco, was that night. Sometimes when they got into a fight, he'd say he was leaving to go to the store to buy some bread and not come back for a week. That's the way it was in the country.

"Come on!" Clara shouted, dragging my mother foot by foot in the icy snow.

My mother was wearing a worn coat and a feeble hat. She didn't have boots; they were too poor. Her tiny feet were covered in her only pair of shoes and a threadbare pair of cotton socks. They were walking in the black of night to her grandmother's one-room log cabin. No electricity, no plumbing. When they arrived, her grandma took one look at my near-frostbit mother and wrapped her in a hand-sewn quilt, warming her beside the hot, black, iron coal stove.

"Her hands and feet are ice," she said, glaring at her daughter.

Many years later, Mom told me that her grandmother never got upset or yelled, but that night her grandma was emphatic: "This child is staying with me. From now on." And from that point on, she did. It turned out that Mom was the lucky one, according to her half siblings. Their mother was mean as a snake and what they would have called back then a rounder. Eventually she'd have five children with four men.

I started fixing when I was in the womb.

By the time I was a six-month-old fetus, I was tuning into my mother constantly, absorbing her emotions like a sponge. When she was excited, I was excited; when she worried, I worried. If she doubted her capacity to be a competent mother, the unborn me was afraid she wasn't going to be able to handle it on her own. I do not know what expectations, conscious or unconscious, my mother conveyed to me in those months. What I do realize now, with insight from years of healing, is that I was a caretaker before I was even born. Early on, my soul enrolled me as little mother. I was to help minimize my mother's angst, keep peace and calm. Make my dad happy. In exchange, I would feel needed and secure in their love. I would be praised and admired for being a "good girl," capably caring for my younger siblings.

As a young girl, my mother was never around babies and never got to hold one. She didn't have a single nurturing gene. When she was a schoolchild, subsisting mostly on beans and bread, and with maybe a nickel every few days to buy a pint of milk, Mom wore the only dress she had every day to school. Yet she flourished in an environment that fed her hunger for learning and achievement. She dreamed of a grander life, had visions of being a court reporter, an airplane pilot, even a doctor. Anything that took her far away from the hollow. Determined to get straight A's, she graduated top of her class from Waverly High and in 1949 landed a secretarial job for the founder of small wholesale paper company in the "big city" Dayton, a hundred miles away. She had a regular paycheck, fashionable suits, a membership at the YWCA. She went out to dinner with charming young professional men with fancy cars. Almost immediately, she set her sights on being a salesperson, what she considered the best job in the company. After all, the salespeople made the most money, got cars, and had expense accounts. Although in 1950 there was only one other female wholesale paper salesperson in the United States, my mother was competitive and driven, and she convinced the president to give her her own territory, where she succeeded in obtaining many new accounts and besting her male counterparts.

Less than two years later, my mother was clear across the country, pregnant and sick, with no support from family or friends and no knowledge of caretaking. I wonder if my mother found herself regretting leaving her successful new career prematurely. Leaving those exciting, carefree days that were all her own.

But my mother was above all a pragmatic student. If she didn't have a clue how to be a mother, she was going to darn sure find out. She picked up some parenting books at the base library and got down to studying, researching, and making lists.

I was born in July 1957 and named Sharmon Ann Hauer, after Sharman Douglas, an American socialite known for her friendship with the British royal family, in particular Princess Margaret. My mother thought the name Sharmon was glamorous and regal, a fitting moniker for her firstborn.

After dinner some evenings, my parents would nestle me in the backseat of their '57 black convertible Thunderbird, alongside their new puppy, a red-haired cocker spaniel named Pretty Thing, and drive down the winding Laguna Canyon Road to Laguna Beach. I was in baby heaven, caressed by the soft, salty sea breeze, my mother and father laughing. They were all mine.

Oh, how I was adored, the center of their universe. For six weeks. And then my mother was pregnant again. Sick again. Suddenly, the nurturing I'd just become accustomed to vanished. Doubled over in nausea and dizziness, Mom left me alone in the living room in my crib while she tried to rest in the bedroom, or she put me on a blanket on the floor with a new toy, hoping I'd be happily distracted. Instead I protested. I did not want her to leave me. I cried in anguish. I never stopped looking for them, hopeful for another loving touch, word, or smile. My craving for my mother's and father's attention mushroomed into an insatiable hunger deep inside me. As the oldest of six children born in rapid succession, I never got to be the baby.

I was ten months old when Michael was born. He was demanding right from the start. Temperamental and fussy, he cried and threw his glass milk bottle against the wall, summoning my mother for another. Exhausted, my mom directed what little energy she had toward him.

Flash forward to 2005. I was in my counselor Lora's home office, a cozy, grandmotherly den with lace doilies on the chair and a brown-and-rust crocheted throw resting on the back of the love seat. The gentle tinkling of water from a tabletop fountain slowed my chattering mind. I sat back in the velour love seat, my eyes closed, listening to her soothing voice.

My best friend, who was becoming an even more devout Catholic and had experienced miraculous emotional healing through a non-denominational prayer process called Theophostics, suggested I try a session. Although I was definitely not a religious person, I was very open spiritually, willing to try all healing modalities. Traditional counseling had gotten me only so far. I figured if I could get out of my own head and have a Theophostics counselor guide an encounter with the Holy Spirit, I'd have a much greater chance of healing the wounds long lodged in my heart.

In our first session, Lora began by saying, "Dear Lord, you have brought Shary here today to heal her wounds and to bring comfort to her heart. Show her the false beliefs and lies that keep her bound. Show her the love that awaits and will free her. In your name, Jesus Christ."

It took me several minutes, almost a half hour, to quiet my wild-monkey mind. *Am I doing this right? God, I'm hungry. Why didn't I eat before I came? I hope we're done by noon or I'll never make my one o'clock.* On and on it went as my body started to feel a contorted energy. My head throbbed with pressure, a pushing and pulling that pulsed behind my left eye and clasped my throat. Random images flashed on the black screen of my inner mind: a giant red fish looking up to the sky, water spouting from its lips like a rainbow fountain. A scary devil's face appeared, and a sense of danger zipped through my body. Suddenly, the devil face flattened, turning into a gorgeous butterfly, resurrected, fluttering away. Near the end of our hour, I saw an image: me. A little girl pulling on a rope, struggling to climb from the depths of a pitch-black cavern. I am scared, tired, crying. *No one is helping me. Someone help me. No one is listening to me. Why is no one ever helping me?*

The next week, in Lora's office, I had a vision of me as a baby, no more than six months old, in a car seat in the back of my dad's T-bird. I was laughing, gurgling, so content. My mom turned around, smiled, and tenderly stroked my tiny hand. My dad pulled into the parking lot of a seaside café. They got out of the car and walked into the restaurant to have lunch. They forgot me. I was in the car alone, the windows rolled up. I started to cry. I cried for a long time. No one heard me. I was going to suffocate from the heat. I was screaming. Gulping for air. Panicking. *Where are they? Why did they leave me? Come back, come back!*

I later learned that the many visions I had over the five months of seeing Lora were not actual memories but representations of trauma I experienced as a child. They were as real as they could be for me. Unlike shadowy dreams, these images were vivid and startling and exposed a singular theme: I felt neglected. Alone. Abandoned.

Even now, it's difficult for me to understand how I, who was raised by good, loving parents in a household where my needs were more than comfortably met, could possibly feel abandoned. To my logical adult self, it feels terribly selfish and whiny to think that I got so tarnished with the emotional and physical residue of abandonment when millions of children actually *were and are* abandoned in such horrific ways.

Yet, after years of exploring my mystical, spiritual realm, I've come to believe that we arrive on this earth with specific soul contracts and that some of us bring the extra luggage of negative energy from emotional suffering accumulated over many lifetimes. I am now convinced that my intense fear of abandonment was energetically linked to my mother's abandonment by her mother.

I was petrified that if I did not step up to help, my mother would desert me. Just as her mother had. Just as her father had.

But this contract came with a stipulation, one that I've come to comprehend only decades later: to be loved in this lifetime, I had to earn it. I had to do something for someone. Caretaking, fixing, and rescuing were the only ways I could receive love. I was not good enough as just Shary. That belief was burned into my DNA and contoured my fifty-seven years in unimaginable ways.

· ·

Life on Brookway Road in Centerville, Ohio, in the late 1950s and the early 1960s, went like this:

When I was ten months old, my brother Mike was born.

When I was twenty months old, my brother Jim was born.

When I was three years old, my brother Bill was born.

I was six and nine when my two sisters were born.

Suddenly and repetitively having to share my parents' love and attention was undoubtedly a difficult adjustment for me. I must have felt replaced and overlooked, dethroned from my position as number one. I wonder if and how I tried to garner my mom and dad's affection those first few years. I know I didn't regress and act like a baby to get their attention. I wasn't disobedient, and I didn't turn aggressive toward my brothers. I only tried to please. But I'm certain that I secretly, maybe not so secretly, began to harbor resentment toward my younger siblings, particularly Mike. Was I already jealous that he was able to get attention by crying, having tantrums, and misbehaving while I had to be the good girl and keep all my anger inside, suffering silently? Dad left for work at eight in the morning, came home for an hour for dinner, and went back to the store until closing at 9:00 p.m. every night. I saw my dad an hour each day. When I heard the garage door go up at six, I'd scamper across the family room and kitchen to greet him at the door. Sunday, his only day off, was busy with going to Mass and getting the car washed, the lawn mowed, and repairs made.

As was typical in the 1960s, my father believed it was his wife's duty to raise the children. But he also relinquished much of the traditional father role: he was not the authority figure, the disciplinarian, the one who set the rules and order of the house. We didn't go to dad for decisions and guidance. He didn't issue punishment, lectures, or lessons. My mom ruled the roost with an iron fist, switch in hand and a yell we all sat up straight for. My dad was the breadwinner, and he was an expert at winning bread. Employed by his father at the Hauer Music Company since he was ten, my father was energetic, creative, and a tireless workaholic who provided a substantial financial kitty to fund our comfortable homes, school tuition, cars, clothing, food, and the essential annual spa (a.k.a. sanity check) getaway for my mother.

By the time I was two years old, I believe I already realized several important truths: (1) my mother was harried; (2) my father was absent; (3) I was to help my mother; and (4) I would have to fend for myself emotionally.

As the oldest and at first the only girl, I was thrust into the role of little helper, the leader of my siblings, a sort of surrogate parent. Still learning how to be responsible for myself, I also needed to be responsible for my brothers. Deferential and dutiful, I watched Mom and followed her around, assisting her whenever I could with her chores—to the other room to find a clean diaper for Mikey or to the crib to entertain Jimmy. I'd mind the boys while Mom took a quick shower and scold them if they got into something that was off-limits. I was an instant babysitter who became protective, maternal, and eventually bossy. Just like my mother.

I wanted desperately to please, to be the perfect child, a reflection of my parents' hopes and dreams. I assumed the classic traits of an oldest child: an overachiever and perfectionist who made a great effort to live up to and exceed my parents' expectations as well as to set a good example for my younger siblings.

By the time I was five, I had already developed the ability to shut down my own feelings—particularly those that were painful. I unconsciously learned to forgo expressing my own sadness, anger, and loneliness. Because there was no one to acknowledge, understand, or console me in the way I needed, my feelings became irrelevant and ultimately repressed. I'd soothe myself by climbing on my beloved brown-and-black rocking horse early mornings, bouncing so hard the horse shimmied clear across the family room floor. In the summer, when no one else in the house was awake, I slipped out to the backyard to swing and sing, aiming my bare toes high to the cloudless sky as I hummed "Baa, Baa, Black Sheep" and "The Farmer in the Dell." My mother, who likely had to suppress her needs for her own mother, raised a daughter who did the same.

My entire life I've turned to others to make me feel of value, to validate my worth. This longing for love that I denied in my early childhood ultimately manifested in my addiction to romance and love. In my twenties, thirties, and forties, I was still a little girl starving for affirmation and desperately clawing for it with a series of men.

When I was six years old, my brother Mikey was five, Jimmy was four, and Billy was three. After Billy was born, my mother took a respite from cranking out newborns by practicing the Catholic-approved rhythm method of birth control. She was able to slow my dad down for almost three years. And get some time to breathe.

But now she was pregnant again. Her hiatus was over. I often wondered what had happened. Did they get out of rhythm? Did my Dad, keen on having seven kids, pressure her? It had to be one or the other, as my mom told me years later that she surely didn't have a burning desire to have more kids. During her upbringing, children were a burden. When she was a young girl, her grandmother could barely scratch a living out of the garden. It took every ounce of energy and every penny to feed and clothe my mother. So it wasn't even in my mom's sphere of thinking that kids were something to eagerly anticipate. It was just a job. It just happened.

My mother was certain she was going to have a girl this time. Her nails were stronger and longer, just as they had been when she was pregnant with me. Years later, my mom admitted to me that she knew she hadn't done it right with me. With another girl, she was hopeful. She wanted another chance to parent well, to give this daughter her attention.

My sister Nancy was born in 1963, and immediately my mother transformed into a completely different mom. *Where did this woman come from?* I wondered. Yes, she had had a three-year break with time to rest and reclaim herself. But my mother seemed unusually happy with Nancy. She called her Nanny Bloom, hugging her close and gazing in her eyes, cooing and bouncing her on her knee as my brown-eyed little sister beamed and gurgled.

What in the world could I have been thinking watching my mother dote on Nancy? That she loved Nancy more than me? Seeing my mother sad and tired and rejecting with me but warm and loving and cheerful with my new sister must have been unbearable.

Much later in my life, a spiritual adviser would tell me that my soul suffered a trauma when I was six. At the time of the consultation, I couldn't recall anything significant happening to me that year. Certainly nothing traumatic. There was a situation with your mother, she said. I'd had a huge disappointment, a trauma that had settled into my cellular memory and informed the rest of my life. Only recently have I come to understand the depth of distress I experienced seeing my mother indulge my baby sister with the love and attention I had been ravenous for. Every inch of me apparently absorbed the shock of rejection and abandonment. I recognize now that losing my mother's love fueled a great unconscious hostility toward myself. I learned to doubt myself, my worth, and I became angry for being defective and flawed. A deep current of hopelessness flowed from that point forward. And unknowingly I also developed a great hostility toward my mother, which I withheld. Or thought I did. I couldn't allow myself to express my anger.

Back then, I swallowed and sucked it up. That's what was expected of me. With so many kids in the family, I was left to my own devices. I didn't demand. I didn't complain. I tried to live up to the one compliment I received from adults—"You are such a good girl"—by appearing far more grown-up and less needy than I really felt.

We lived in a mushrooming new suburb, Centerville, with new brick ranch homes, surrounded by other white, middle-class families with lots of kids.

With a teeming creek behind our house and more than fifty acres of woods and open field at the end of Brookway Road, we had endless freedom to roam and play. In the summer, my brothers and their friends left the house early in the morning with bows and arrows and fishing poles, and returned by dinner—always served promptly at 6:00 p.m. when my dad got home. We rode our bikes and walked everywhere, and our parents did not give a thought to worry about us. We had absolute respect for authority at school and at home.

To transport us to school and church, we had every configuration of the Ford Country Squire woodie station wagon, the practical and only car to tote our growing family. Every year, the week before school, my mother took us to J. C. Penney at the Town and Country shopping center, where each of us got a new supply of white cotton underwear, navy socks, and school shoes. Except me. My feet were too wide, and there were no shoes at Penney's to fit. Every year my mom had to make a special trip to Roderer Shoes to order a new pair of Buster Browns or penny loafers.

In our home, caretaking—feeding and sheltering—equaled love. My parents never hugged or kissed. I don't remember hearing them speak kind and loving words to each other. It was all business. The only time I heard "I love you" was when my mom sent me a big pink fancy card with lace from Florida when I was eight years old. "Happy Valentine's Day," it read. "I love you." I studied those words, reading them over and over again in disbelief. I wanted so much for it to be true.

Not until I was in my forties and in another round of therapy did the concept of "childhood neglect" surface. I had never considered that I and my siblings had been neglected. I always thought that neglected kids were parentless or abused or hungry or homeless or living in horrific, unsafe conditions. I didn't realize parents could emotionally neglect their children. I learned that inadequate attention to a child's emotional needs—her need for affection—and a lack of emotional support constitute emotional neglect. I didn't realize that emotional neglect could be as dangerous to a child's well-being as physical neglect is to a child's health and safety—that it can lead to poor self-image, alcohol or drug abuse, other destructive behaviors, or, as in my case, love addiction.

· ·

In 1966, when I was nine, my sister Patsy was born. Whatever little sense of childhood freedom, play, and wonder I still had was now sacrificed. I was Patsy's second mother, watching her, changing her diapers, dressing her.

There is an old thirty-five-millimeter slide of us six kids sitting on the edge of the pool at a motel in Indian Rocks Beach, on our first family trip to Florida for Easter break, in 1967. It was a cloudless sunny day and our eyes squinted as we looked toward Dad's camera. My towheaded brothers, Jimmy and Billy, seven and six, sat to the right of me. At ten years old, I sat in the middle of the lineup, with Patsy, just fourteen months old, perched in my lap. Next to me was Nancy, nearly four. Mikey, almost nine, was a different shade of brown than the rest of us, the sun turning him almost cocoa black. I was just ten months older than Mikey but was twenty-five pounds heavier and six inches taller. I looked like I could be my siblings' mother or aunt, not their sister. I was the only one not smiling.

It must have seemed like the zillionth time I had to watch my brothers and sisters. Especially Patsy. She was still a baby. She couldn't swim. But she wanted to, desperately, and scampered to the edge of the pool over and over again. Each time I ran to grab her and placed her back on the lounge chair with a stern warning. She cried and screamed and kicked me mercilessly. How I wanted to get away from all of this, to be on the beach collecting colorful shells. How I wished I could have been carefree like other ten-year-olds. To play when I wanted to, cry and scream when I felt like it, snuggle close to my dad when I needed a hug. I wouldn't worry about anything. Nothing at all. I would be free to let my thoughts wander wherever they wanted to go. I would ask my mom if she could take me places more often. And I wouldn't feel bad or selfish. If my mom and dad asked me to do something and I didn't want to do it, I could say no and not fear what they would say. I wouldn't have to watch Patsy every minute to make sure she didn't crawl into anything dangerous or worry about what kind of trouble my brother Mike was getting into. It wouldn't matter.

I'd care about only me. What made me happy. What made me sad. What I wanted. What I needed more of. I could talk a lot more and express how I really felt inside rather than holding back so much. I could go off to the creek and play a long time without thinking about what time I'd have to be back home. I would laugh a lot more and draw and paint—not just with crayons and coloring books but with real paint on real art paper. My mom would hang my creations on the refrigerator door because they would be so beautiful. She'd tell me how pretty the colors were and ask me how I came up with the designs. She'd look at me and listen carefully as I described how a bunch of purple hyacinths just came to me. She'd tell me how artistic I was and hug me close and say, "You're so special. How talented you are in so many ways. I am so proud of you. Do you know that?" I'd smile really big and say, "Yes, I'm very talented" and would feel so happy inside.

I realize now that I was a joyless and empty girl with an edge of sadness about me all the time. I didn't have the experience of being a child—spontaneous, fun, and foolish. I silently cried out, scrounging to be filled with any sort of affection or attention, some recognition or acknowledgment from my parents. When I didn't receive it, I withdrew further into myself, stifling and denying my frustration and sadness. I couldn't go to my mom and dad to tell them about my troubles; they had no time to listen. Not until I was nearly forty, when I was diagnosed with chronic clinical depression, did I realize that I had been depressed since childhood. I had been mute, suffering in silence, like all good girls did.

• ☙ •

Every Easter I would get my own pink basket that my mother had wrapped in volumes of shiny pink cellophane. The basket would have pink plastic grass filled with an amazing assortment of pastel foil-wrapped chocolate eggs, chocolate bunnies, and marshmallow Peeps. Maybe a small toy or two would be tucked inside that messy grass. And not only did I get a basket from Mom and Dad, but we also collected baskets from Grandma and Grandpa, whose house we went to for Easter Sunday dinner. Their sixteen grandchildren would be presented with baskets filled to the brim with more elegant chocolates and even bigger bunnies.

Easter was my favorite holiday because I got to feel special, like I mattered. Two weeks before Easter, one day a year, I was invited to go shopping with my grandma for an Easter outfit. I adored my grandmother, the only person in my life who in my young girl's eyes personified love. And she was mine for a day! Grandma would pull into our driveway on Brookway Road in her long, black Cadillac Eldorado for the thirty-minute drive to Rike's department store in downtown Dayton.

She looked so tiny driving her big, black tank, rigid, ten inches from the back of the seat with both of her gloved hands planted on the inner-tube-sized steering wheel. I knew we were getting close when I inhaled the luscious, yeasty smells of bread baking at the Wonder Bread factory on South Patterson Boulevard.

"Watch out for the cops," she'd say before she turned the wrong way down the narrow one-way alley to the parking lot behind Grandpa's store. I didn't know why she said it, but I obeyed, looking to my left and then my right, worried that something bad might happen if I didn't.

Before shopping, we'd go to the Coin Room on the second floor, the fancy dining room with what seemed like a hundred tables and glowing crystal chandeliers, to have lunch at a table with white linen. I loved watching the elegant women wearing hats and pearls lunching, their conversations animated but hushed. I wanted to be a little lady, mindful of placing the cloth napkin on my lap and holding the heavy silverware just so. Grandma would ask me about school and friends and other things, but I was so shy. I don't know if I said much.

The shopping itself was horrendous. Painful. I was a fat—we used to say chubby—girl. So I couldn't fit into the clothes made for girls, and we'd always have to go to the ladies' department. As a ten-year-old girl, shopping for dresses in the ladies' department was humiliating. But Grandma made it tolerable. She never uttered a condescending or critical word, never made me feel fat or inferior. She was kind and gentle and simply had a job to do. She knew where she had to go to get something to fit me. As a professional seamstress in her younger days, she could transform anything into a wearable frock. And we shopped not only for a new dress but for a coordinating coat, for I always needed a coat for church on typically chilly Easter Sunday mornings. And we bought white gloves and new patent-leather shoes. To cap off our day, I got to go to Grandma's home with her to have dinner.

After stopping at the butcher, we'd pull into her garage on Tait Road by 4:00 p.m. Grandma would put the chicken in the refrigerator, offer me a bottle of cold 7UP and pretzels, and shoot straight down to her basement sewing machine to get started renovating my dress and coat. I'd sit at the dining room table painting horses or a vase of daisies with the paint-by-numbers kit Grandma had let me pick out in the toy department after our dress shopping. Two hours later, I'd help her with dinner by setting the table, rolling the Pillsbury crescent rolls on the baking sheet, and preparing a plate of Grandpa's favorite dessert, cherry Jell-O. How I relished the time alone with Grandma and Grandpa, as they always wanted to know more about me, asking me about my teachers, my grades, if I wanted another helping—as if I were the most important person in the world.

3
The Dance of Denial

August 16, 1989

I did not hear John come up the stairs. I must have been in a deep sleep. He turned on the bathroom light. I thought I was dreaming. I untangled my legs from the sheets and lifted my head off the pillow. The digital clock blinked a red 1:03 a.m. in the darkness. His flight from Copenhagen must have been delayed; he was supposed to be home by ten. I turned and looked up. He stood by the bed, briefcase in hand, suit jacket still on.

"Hi," I mumbled. "Welcome home."

"I don't love you anymore. I want a divorce." Thud. My chest clenched. I struggled to breathe.

"What? What are you talking about?"

"I'm unhappy. I've been unhappy," he said. "We're different. Everything is different now."

I sunk down in the bed and covered myself with the blanket, willing his voice—the night—away.

"What's different?" I managed to ask.

"You don't like the rides at Kings Island. You don't like to watch sports or throw parties."

This could not be happening. This was not supposed to happen. We are married. For life. Forever.

"I feel like we're just friends, just roommates. That's all we are."

"Rides at King's Island? That's why you want a divorce?" I asked.

"I'm tired. Long flight. I'm going downstairs to sleep," he said.

37

I was too stunned to respond. Even if I could have mustered the words, what would I have said? I never questioned. I never fought back. He never listened. That was our pattern.

I lay awake, unable to process, and only thin thoughts of *he's just tired* and *we just need to have some time together* seeped in, attempting to drown out the panic gasping in my throat. In the days that followed, I traipsed to work and home again like a zombie. It was as if in the exact moment of John's pronouncement, a magnitude 9.0 earthquake had convulsed my body and spirit, irreparably dismantling my inner landscape. Vivacious, lovable, and optimistic Shary was now a shapeless, colorless amoeba struggling to make it upstream.

Far worse than blindsiding me was his refusal to discuss it. Discuss us. At all. No explanation, no "We'll talk about it later," no expression of regret, no "I'm sorry." When I tried to broach the subject, he slammed the door in my face. He would not allow another word about "us." In the rare moments he was home, I searched his face, his eyes for a hint of sadness or softness. Instead, my husband of five years was a cold, mute stranger. I wanted my ceaseless crying to end. I wanted him to hold me and tell me he wanted to work on us, that everything would be okay. I wanted to know that every couple has the five-year itch. We'd get through ours stronger and more in love. I wanted to shake him and scream in his face, "No. We. Are. Not. Quitting. We are going to do it my way now." I wanted to curl up and play possum so the nightmare would end. I wanted to see our children—laughing, fishing in our backyard cove. All of these things. I was tormented.

Yet I could not express any of this to him. If I yelled and screamed or cried, he wouldn't have acknowledged me. He would have walked away. He would shut things—shut me—down instantly. My anguish was unbearable. Echoes of my childhood—feeling neglected, unheard, and invisible—reverberated in my barren heart. And now my ultimate terror, abandonment, was barreling toward me.

August 25, 1989

The next week, in a psychologist's office on the fourteenth floor overlooking downtown Columbia, John sat expressionless, rigid in the chair. I sat five feet away, numb but optimistic.

"Do you want to work on your marriage?" the therapist asked.

"Of course I do," I said.

"There's nothing to work on," John said.

Thirty minutes. That's all it took. I didn't realize it then. John had agreed to go to one counseling session only to convince me that our relationship was unsalvageable. He was dead set on getting a divorce. But it didn't register. My fortress of denial was impenetrable. Thirty-two years of walls guarded my heart. I was simply unable to accept that my dream was imploding.

"John is one of the most serious cases I have ever seen," the psychologist told me the next day when I called. "He is so cold, icy. No, he's never coming back."

I couldn't fight, I couldn't suggest, I couldn't say. I didn't have a say, a voice. He wouldn't talk, he wouldn't listen, he wasn't there. No healing, no treatment sought. Death sentence to execution in ten days.

September 13, 1989

I arrived home at 7:00 p.m. after a two-and-a-half-hour flight from Dayton, tired and hungry but happy that my interview for a new corporate job had gone well. Two weeks earlier, out of the blue, NCR's human resources vice president had called to tell me I was a candidate for a director role in a highly visible new division at NCR's world headquarters in Dayton. While I was intent on saving my hemorrhaging marriage, the opportunity to flee, return to Ohio, and sequester myself in the comfort of my childhood home felt like an act of God, an absolute miracle.

Besides, we were barely coexisting. He came home every night after ten and went straight to the guest room over our garage. In the few moments I saw him the previous week, I mentioned that I was headed to Dayton for an interview. "That's great," he said. "You deserve it." He didn't even look up. His voice was flat and indifferent.

I was the leading candidate, the VP told me. Finally, a sliver of hope poking out of the morass of gloom. I wasn't thinking about the future, the next steps with John, where I'd live long term, even what the new job would entail. All I knew was that I needed to escape from my hell, and here was a possible lifeline.

When I went to the refrigerator to grab a can of Tab and a sand-wich, I saw a box of half-eaten pizza and three wine coolers. That's odd. John was a beer drinker. The last thing he'd touch was a straw-berry wine cooler. And the pizza box was from a hole-in-the-wall joint miles away, on the other side of town.

"What's all this?" I asked him, as he walked into the kitchen, his arms loaded with a fresh supply of dress shirts and trousers he just emptied from our bedroom closet.

He pretended not to hear me.

"The wine coolers and pizza. Did you have a party?"

"Just thought you'd like them. That's all."

I drank a cooler only now and then. He knew it wasn't my favorite, and I rarely touched pizza. Yet I wanted to believe him. I wanted to believe that he still cared about and loved me, especially when I was away.

"Thank you," I said as I made my way upstairs to change out of my business suit.

September 22, 1989

Hurricane Hugo made landfall in Charleston, South Carolina, as a ferocious category 4 storm with 120 mile-per-hour winds. That night it weakened just barely before mowing down forests of long-leaf pines on its way to Columbia.

I was scared. It was my first hurricane. And I was alone. John was traveling. At work, it was all anyone could talk about all week: what stores still had lumber on the shelves, who had the best prices on bottled water, where the most rollicking hurricane parties were going to be, how much liquor to buy. That night I lay in bed shaking as the wind roared throughout the night. Our huge paned windows rattled and shrieked. Sheets of heavy rain beat sideways against the house.

John called early the next morning from New York to see if I was okay. I was instantly uplifted, as if the storm of the previous thirty-seven days had passed and the healing sun was beaming down only on me. *He was worried about me. He cares for me. He still wants me.*

September 29, 1989

The human resources vice president called to offer me the position—a promotion and sizable salary increase to be the new director of strategic marketing at headquarters in Dayton. I was thrilled to have something new to dive into, to distract me.

One week later, lugging two suitcases stuffed with business suits, I evacuated and set up camp in my old bedroom at my parent's home. I started my new job a week after our fifth wedding anniversary. Discombobulated and shattered inside, I summoned the energy to suit up in the morning to look crisp and perky. When old friends and curious colleagues asked about our new long-distance arrangement, I laughed it off.

"Oh, he'll be back up here in no time. You know John, always gunning for a promotion," I said.

Naturally, I was the consummate professional, conducting meetings and conference calls with a confident edge, until I slipped off to the ladies' room around the corner to silently sob. At night I'd barely say hello to my worried parents before retreating to my canopied bed. Number 2 pencil in hand and a pile of yellow-lined paper, I started a makeshift journal, ranting and wailing, emotions torpedoing out of me, searing the pages. Night after night, this was my new routine: I thrashed on the page, voraciously consumed self-help books, and cried myself to a fitful sleep.

Two months into my private hell, I decided I needed talk to someone who could help make sense of this and him, someone wise who could comfort and guide me. I reluctantly called the company's Employee Assistance Hotline to make an appointment with a counselor. A week later, I met with a diminutive psychotherapist, a Dr. Ruth look-alike who wore a heavy-knit, maroon cardigan and black orthopedic shoes.

"Aren't you feeling rage? Don't you want to hurt him? Get revenge?" she asked. Her meek features suddenly animated.

"I'm angry, I'm sad, but I don't want revenge."

"When my husband left me twenty-three years ago, I had a dream that he was sitting in a chair, his arms and legs tied," she said. "Above him was a huge, heavy, sharp, shiny blade—a guillotine." Her eyes

41

narrowed and she became more excited. "The guillotine was released, and the blade flew down on him in an instant, chopping off his penis." She smiled.

I squirmed in my chair and looked at my watch. My mother was right. She'd always been suspicious of psychiatrists, telling me they were loopy and had far more issues than their patients could ever dream of.

"I don't want to chop off his penis. I just want him to come back."

January 1990

Throughout our separation and divorce proceedings, John was in Dayton frequently for meetings. I panicked at the thought of seeing him. Yet I wanted to, desperately. I hoped to sense a hint of love in his eyes. I needed to hear possibility in his "Hi" as he strolled past the cubicles in that upbeat, gregarious way of his, like a politician in a victory parade.

Five hundred miles between Dayton and Columbia, and still there was no way I could escape John's presence. How was I to accept us splitting up when his name, his voice, he himself seemed to be always around? How could I move on with my life when I saw him in the cafeteria standing a hundred feet away and could barely walk back upstairs, shaking, trembling, and sweating so much?

My torture was magnified tenfold because we had to work together. Once again, my department worked closely with his, and I felt responsible for maintaining friendly working relations. What would the bosses and our colleagues say if we were not talking to one another? If we were outwardly hostile? In meeting after meeting with John, I had to turn the "on" switch on, playing the role of affable, supportive teammate while stuffing my wretched knot of anxiety, despair, and hope. God, it was exhausting.

On the home front, I was still in fixing mode, even managing the divorce I was dead set against. I resented having to find the lawyer to handle our divorce. He wanted the divorce. Why didn't *he* get a fucking lawyer? Why didn't I fight it? Stall indefinitely? Did I feel it was inevitable, that I had no choice but to proceed? He knew I would take care of everything. I always did. I wanted to sue him for divorce. But my lawyer, an intelligent and sympathetic woman, convinced me that there was no advantage in suing John. I was a career woman making a good salary, and we were childless. No judge was going to award me alimony. A dissolution was the best, most expedient course, she advised.

For the most part, we agreed on how to divide our property. I took the furniture I came in with; he got his. I took my lovely antique cathedral-style maple armoire, and he got to keep the cheap sandbox of a waterbed. He kept the Audi; I kept my BMW. He got the boat, which turned out to be in the shop more than in the water. I got the bulk of our paltry investments. He got the house.

Even when we met at Arby's for lunch on a gray, below-freezing January day to sign the initial dissolution papers, I was hopeful he'd reconsider. In the back of my romanticized mind, I wanted to hear, "You know, I thought about this, about us, about the last five years a lot over the holidays. I've decided not to sign these."

Standing behind him in line to order, I attempted to rustle pleasant memories, laughing about a tired-looking miniature Christmas tree stationed by the condiments. He turned around. His eyes glared at the side of my face. "God, look at all that gray hair," he said, pointing to the new silver strands framing my face.

We sat down at a table in the corner. He looked at the papers, turned to the last one, and signed it quickly as he gulped his sandwich.

Thwack. Another body blow. My eyes started to fill with tears. I couldn't look at him. "I never thought you'd go ahead with this. I hoped you'd change your mind."

"I don't want to be married anymore," he said.

Silent, defeated, I slogged wearily to the parking lot. He got into his car. I swore I saw a smile on his face as he drove away.

Even though it had been five months since John had said he wanted out, I could not yet see or face my reality. I could not see that I kept setting myself up for continual slaps in the face from John. Hoping for a sign of warmth and kindness, I instead got terse, impatient, frosty John. My husband who didn't want to be my husband anymore. Who had no qualms about proclaiming so. Those slaps stung so hard that I couldn't function in the afternoon. They were the kind that lingered like a heavy fog, slumping over me for days.

I had no idea back then that I created and perpetuated my own suffering or that for six years, I'd gone overboard caretaking, cheerleading and loving John too much. Now that our demise was inevitable, I was panicking. I clutched the dream of "us" for dear life and could not let go—which only accelerated John's distancing. But I didn't know any of that. All I understood was that love always equaled anguish. The greater the love, the deeper the anguish.

February 21, 1990

Somehow I was able to find humor in my suffering by laughing at the fact that I was literally and figuratively falling apart. One week, a back molar broke in half. My hair was coming out in clumps. The shower drain was clogged, and the hair that remained on my head was turning grayer by the day. It was almost white, with a baby-powder pallor, a deadly cast to it. And another tooth cracked and fell out over the weekend. That same week, I had another reminder of my past life with John. I ran into Sandy, the wife of a colleague and friend, Ron Scott, in the hallway, and she said, "Oh, I'm so sorry to hear about you two. I thought you were so perfect for one another."

So did I.

March 6, 1990

As the court date for our dissolution hearing loomed, I woke up in the middle of the night ready to scream. I could not yet resolve my anger and shock about the way our marriage was coming to an end. Our "big day" was just a week away. All during the prior seven months I had expected to have an opportunity to sit down to discuss our feelings like two adults before we formally severed our vows. Instead, more anger and bitterness made a home in my heart. I knew I would eventually accept that John wanted a divorce. But I was simply unprepared for his alienation. To obliterate a six-year relationship without discussion was unbearable. I would not get the resolution and closure I needed. I was following orders, essentially a soldier obediently marching off to a war I was vehemently opposed to. Gutted, lifeless, the all of me felt split open, splayed, and nailed to a bloody plank.

More than once I begged God for answers in my expanding journal: "WHY, WHY, WHY? What is the purpose of this endless torture?" Through the haze of tears, I could barely breathe, torment stabbing my gut. "Tell me, God, why . . . ?" I scrawled. All I could feel was the seething hell of abandonment. I couldn't see out of it. I was an adult functioning in a very adult corporate setting, but emotionally I was a three-year-old, drowning in the hovering doom of having to be alone. The one time I thought of suicide was then. Although I didn't seriously contemplate ending my life, I was inconsolable, pleading to God for my despair to end. "Take me now," I sobbed more than once. Twenty-one years later, my intuitive adviser, Marcella, was able to read the devastation the divorce had wreaked. "You had a trauma, a soul split, an opportunity 'to go,'" she said. "Not a suicide. But you hit a chasm. You stopped. Your life stopped. You fell into an abyss. You had to climb out on your own. It was very traumatizing."

March 9, 1990

I hated all the signs of not being a couple: our phone message recorder, which had said, "Shary and I aren't home right now," now said, "I'm away right now." And the return labels on packages of my mail forwarded by his assistant Ginger no longer read "Shary and John Gray," just "John Gray." The vanishing vestiges of our life together tore me apart.

March 13, 1990

Our dissolution hearing on March 13 in the Common Pleas Court of Montgomery County, Ohio, took all of five minutes. We stood four feet apart in front of the judge and nodded when he asked if we agreed to the terms of the decree. We signed the papers, and we walked out. We were officially divorced.

"Have fun in Florida," he said, before jumping in his car and driving back to the office. Two hours later, I flew to a spa in Fort Lauderdale with my mother to sit in a daze and bake in the sun like a sphinx, hoping to begin thawing my frozen heart.

March 21, 1990

"I'll pack up your stuff and send it to you. It will be too painful for you to come back here," John said on the phone.

"No, I'm coming down. I'll be there next Sunday," I said.

I had found the perfect home, a charming 1938 Tudor a half mile from my parents, in the Hills and Dales neighborhood in which I had grown up. With dozens of big oaks and maples; apple, cherry, and peach trees; a garden of heirloom roses; flowering magnolias; and its original greenhouse, this place felt like a cozy and cheerful nest, a place to rejuvenate my weary, battered spirit. Brimming with character, it had rich wood floors and a grand fireplace in the loft living room, a winding staircase that led to my alcove bedroom, and an outrageous green-and-Pepto-Bismol-pink-tiled bathroom. Finally, a home I would call mine. There would be no pleasing anyone but myself. My own healing sanctuary.

March 28, 1990

I flew to Columbia on Sunday morning, and nervously waited for John to pick me up at the baggage claim. Here I was again, at ground zero, filled with familiar yet strange, conflicting emotions. The mechanical (in-denial) me was all business, calm and ready to split our assets, officially divide our lives. The heart-centered (real) me, was hurting and hopeful. Maybe he'll get nostalgic and reconsider the divorce when he sees all the boxes stacked up for the movers.

"Hi," he said, picking up my bag and tossing it in the backseat of his Audi.

"Hey." He looked good. He had lost some weight and was sun-tanned—he'd probably been out enjoying the boat as much as possible. That was it. Our reunion conversation had concluded. He tore right into comfortable territory: work and updating me on all of the corporate dragons he was slaying.

We went straight to our house so I could begin preparing for the movers, who were coming Tuesday. I had hours ahead of me, having to go through every drawer and closet to pull my belongings aside and label them. I opened up the refrigerator to grab a bottle of cold water when my hand skimmed a bright blue-and-white plate with pink flowers covered in plastic wrap. It wasn't our plate. I turned up a corner of the wrap to see a homemade dinner of steak, potatoes, and green beans.

"Who made you dinner?" I asked.

He walked away and turned the TV on.

"Oh, Ginger felt sorry for me. Thought I was going to starve." Ginger was married. I knew it wasn't her doing. She didn't cook, and she certainly wasn't the motherly type.

I started in the kitchen, opening cabinet after cabinet, emptying most of the pots and pans and bakeware. It was tedious having to inventory every drinking glass, mug, and gadget.

"What about this apple corer?" His mom had given it to us. "Do you want it?" I said. He was lying on the couch watching a basketball game.

"No, keep it," he said.

I'll never get through all this at this rate, I thought. I had five more rooms to go, plus several boxes in the garage to sort through. I sped the process along by ignoring the silverware drawer, pantry, and small appliance cabinet. He can have it all, I decided before moving upstairs.

About 6:00 p.m., after the game was over, John asked me if I wanted to go to dinner at Rusty Anchor, a new seafood restaurant lakeside. "That sounds great," I said, and I went to change and spruce up a bit. We got into his car for the short drive down Johnson Marina Road.

"What's this? I asked, picking up what looked like a makeup bag from the passenger-seat pocket. Silence. I opened the worn fake-leather pouch.

"I don't know how that got there."

"What do you mean you don't know?"

"God, you're here for only four hours and already you're abusing me."

His typical response. Over the previous several months, when I had attempted to talk about us, he'd snap back with, "I don't need any more aggravation" or "Don't abuse me." And just like that, he would shut down any further talk.

I didn't know how to push. Actually, I was afraid to push. I avoided conflict at all costs, intent on keeping things peaceful. And I knew with John, I'd always lose. It wasn't worth the energy. So I tiptoed, just as I had as a little girl, silent and compliant, tucking all of the agony deep inside.

May 17, 1990

It had been nine months since he had said he wanted a divorce and I was still obsessing about John. I kept having thoughts about him calling, stopping by my office, or asking me to dinner. I wrenched myself wondering what he was doing, who he was with, whether he thought about me, whether he felt any sadness or regret. I still cried. Every night during the week. On the weekend several times a day. I was depressed, sleepless, exhausted, nauseous, unable to fathom why my pain continued to feel so real, so recent, so fresh. Nine months of a miserable existence, and I wondered how much longer it would continue. If I could bear it. I was going through withdrawal but did not yet know that. I did not comprehend that my addiction to John and the dream of "us" was as powerful and debilitating as heroin.

Despite my encounter with the smiling guillotine psychologist, I started seeing a new therapist.

July 8, 1990

I was in my office on a phone call with our New York advertising agency when John sauntered in unannounced and plopped down in one of my chairs. It wasn't the first time he'd done that. As usual, the conversation was 90 percent work related and 120 percent John-focused. We talked for thirty minutes about his mom and dad coming the following week. I complimented him on his attractive gray pin-striped suit and royal purple tie—why did I still flatter that asshole? He detailed his search for his next position, and on and on he went. I wondered what it would be like to finally stand up to him. When would I be brash enough to say, "I don't have time right now" or "I'm not interested in talking about your life. I have to deal with my own concerns" or, more to the truth, "Who the hell do you think you are coming in here? After all that you've done, all that I've put up with and you still have the audacity to walk in here as if nothing has happened?

Do not come in here again. I do not want to see you in my office ever again."

August 25, 1990

I had a resolution dream. I was in our home in Columbia, packing kitchen items into cardboard boxes. John and I were talking when he finally revealed the truth: yes, he had started seeing someone before we got divorced. Yes, he had been seeing her when we were married. Yes, there had been others during our marriage.

October 23, 1990

As if the gods were using all their power to keep me from moving on with my life, I was back in Columbia for a few days, this time at his plant overseeing a video production, which meant working with several of his direct reports, all of whom I knew and enjoyed. I was determined to be nonchalant and all business. Thankfully, John and I managed to avoid each other most of the day. But at nights, on his way out the door, he'd make a point of stopping by my visitor's cubicle to say goodnight, and I'd perked up inside. We'd chat politely about the latest takeover talk and the newest restaurants in town. How sad, I thought, that we hadn't or wouldn't or couldn't ever dive below the surface to have a personal discussion about our actual feelings. We were stuck in a pattern, unable to shake free.

People were amazed how well we got along, whether in Columbia or Dayton.

"I never would have expected you two to carry on like you do," one of our associates said.

Oh yes, I thought. *Isn't it wonderful that we both pretend so well?* I continued to force myself to play the role of detached coworker while I grieved silently. I thought I had no choice. How else was I to cope?

November 15, 1990

Finally, after fourteen months, I felt the heavy cloak of pain and denial begin to lift. I was enjoying my new home, new friends, a blind date, fun with my little nieces and nephew, and I was going back to get my master's degree. More promising was that I started to get a glimpse of John through a different lens, a more accurate lens: he was boring. He was consumed with himself, his work, his reputation. Somewhere in my consciousness, I started to get the sense that I wanted and deserved more.

But I still cried. I still hung on. I still loved him. I still directed an inordinate amount of my thinking hours to him, worrying about his health with his constant travel and the stress of his demanding role. I still dreamed of John, either reconciling with me or sitting with me calmly, telling me how he was going to change. I could not let go.

November 23, 1990

After work on a Friday, I met my good friend and work buddy Bill for drinks at the Marriott, across the street from the office. We found a cozy spot in the dark lounge, ordered a glass of merlot and a Budweiser, grabbed a basket of freshly popped popcorn, and settled in for an overdue evening of laughs and work talk. Moments later, John walked in. He saw me immediately, nodded, and crossed the room to join some of his teammates. *Good,* I thought, *he'll be far enough away that I won't have to hear him.* That didn't stop him from coming over to join in our conversation several times.

Why did he have to say, "Jim [his boss] asked me last week why you and I couldn't get back together again. He wants you to come back to Columbia so we can get our product promotions on the right track"?

And later: "Wouldn't Lew—the colleague we had dinner with in Columbia the night John told me to prepare a "baby business plan"—freak out if I brought you with me to his house for dinner on Saturday?"

Didn't he know that those sorts of things, which just rolled off his tongue, sent me into a tailspin? I'd be haunted by them for days, analyzing his every word, dissecting for evidence that he still cared for me. What did he mean by that? How did he respond when Jim suggested we get back together? My spinning was endless. And was that the point? Did he lob these ticklers at me for his amusement, to see how I'd react? To torture me?

Who knows what his motives were? I could barely understand

mine. All I knew was that I was operating on a primeval instinct. Despite the fact that we had been divorced for eight months and lived in separate states and separate homes, despite the sprouting inklings that I was ready to move on, John was still my sun. I still orbited around him. No gravitational force could pull me away. I was so desperately fearful of being alone that I clung to the one source of love and attention that I had counted on. I stayed enslaved in a delusion that just maybe he'd come back. Without a man by my side, I felt I was not worth loving. I was incomplete, empty, meaningless. Superwoman with her kryptonite. Diminished and powerless.

January 29, 1991

I called Ginger to thank her for forwarding another box of my mail from Columbia.

"John's sure up in Dayton a lot lately. Is he ever there?" I said.

"He'll probably keep coming back and forth until she graduates," she said.

Click. Click. Click. In rapid gunfire order, all the signs suggesting there was someone else pierced into a single clear image.

The co-op student. I gulped.

"Oh, that's right," I said. "Remind me of her name again."

"Maria."

Flash. A laser beam of searing light walloped me out of my two-year daze.

It turned out that Maria, one of his employees, was the one he was having an affair with. Maria was the one he dismissed me for. Maria, a skinny and plain co-op student from the University of South Carolina with dirty blond hair, who at twenty years old was thirteen years younger than John.

She was the one who called our house one early Saturday morning six months after we moved to Columbia.

"Is John there?" I heard a meek Southern girl's voice on the other end. I handed the phone to John and he mumbled something like, "I'll call you later. . . ."

"Who was that?"

"Oh, nobody. Some co-op student at the office working on our presentation."

"What does she want?"

"Nothing." She was the one who slept in our bed and ate her breakfast in our cozy windowed nook overlooking Lake Murray just days after I fled to Dayton. The one who liked greasy pizza and sickeningly sweet strawberry wine coolers. The one who apparently needed heavy spackling, given the duffel-sized makeup bag I found in his car. The one who surely had her family over for dinner to show off her new boyfriend—an executive!—and his beautiful home on the lake, all of them laughing, ebullient with wine, sitting in our dining room with the rich traditional cherrywood chairs and table that I loved and had special-ordered after months of searching.

In almost two years, I had been unable, unwilling to face the truth, to connect the dots. I believed him. He always worked hard, traveled a lot, never had time for anything but work. He always made it sound like his head was reeling, overwhelmed with the responsibilities of overseeing the company's biggest new product launch in five years. I believed him when I asked him that August night, when he said he wanted out of our marriage, "Is there another woman?"

"No, I wish there was. Wouldn't it be easier that way?"

I believed him. *Good ol' trusting Shary. She'll never know.* What a fool I'd been. Everyone else must have known for months, probably over a year. I was humiliated. The evidence had been there all along. But I ignored it, stubbornly harboring fantasies of our future. I was delusional and addicted and would not relinquish hope until I had no choice.

I had vowed my whole heart when we were married in 1984. But I realized he had come to our partnership only halfway, if that. He lied, misled, deceived for six years. The truth was, he had been ambivalent about us even after our first year of marriage and had gradually grown more distant until his distance became actual infidelity. He was a fraud. A coward of the highest order who never once had the decency to utter, "I'm sorry." Not one time. He misled me in my hopes for our future, allowing me to go on talking about babies when he knew there would be none.

Despite my burning anger and agonizing hurt, I never blamed John. I knew I was not the victim. Ultimately, I knew I had been responsible too. I'd fallen for a married man whose five-year marriage had dissolved in part because of me. He'd again fallen for another woman, and our five-year marriage imploded. As I sensed John straying, I sharpened my talons, grappling for more attention, overwhelming him in my frenzied attempts to enmesh him permanently. I had lied, misled, and deceived myself.

It seemed that many, perhaps most aspects of our life together were a show, just a cover-up. I wonder now: was *any* of it real? What a fantasy I lived in. A charade. After replaying the same scenes over for twenty-five years, I see now that our marriage was a dance. I entered the relationship in a fog of fantasy, high on the euphoria of being seduced by a strong and charismatic prince. I played the role of the needy, selfless pleaser and fixer, and John played the charming, selfish taker and controller. And we called it love. Our dance unfolded flawlessly, unconsciously. John maintained the lead and I followed. To the bitter end.

With John, my cocooned addiction to love and romance roared to life, accelerated, and defined my next twenty years.

4
Resurrection

The week before Christmas 1990, eleven months after my divorce, AT&T launched a hostile takeover bid to acquire NCR, the company where I had worked for eight years. AT&T had been on the hunt to enhance its computer capabilities and targeted NCR as the perfect match. But NCR's executive team and board were vehement in their opposition to AT&T's overture and immediately assembled a team to combat the takeover attempt. The vice president of corporate communications tapped me to serve on special assignment to the communications and PR team. Corporate takeovers were typically played out in the public relations forum, so this new team was going to be in the crosshairs of our fight. I was elated to be handpicked for such a visible and important role and thrilled to temporarily step away from my strategic marketing role, which had become maddeningly unchallenging.

Ensconced in my interim office, a spacious cubicle facing huge windows overlooking NCR's Old River Park, I set up camp. Twice daily we powwowed with our New York City–based lawyers and PR firm, crafting our media messages, creating ads to run in *The New York Times* and *The Wall Street Journal,* and playing defense against AT&T's massive army of takeover big guns. I served as an NCR spokesperson, playing tough and evasive with the national and local media, who were hungry for a juicy Goliath consumes David story.

One afternoon in early March, one of my colleagues, Dick, the genteel, silver-haired director of community relations, knocked on my cubicle door.

"Did you know you have a new member of your fan club?" Dick said. "Patrick was falling all over himself to see and meet you the other day. I gave him your name and office number. I hope that was okay."

I chuckled. Several work buddies who knew the details of my breakup with John were on the lookout for potential suitors for me. According to Dick, Patrick was a young NCR salesman based out of the Dayton office. That's all I knew about him.

Two days later, Patrick called, introduced himself, and invited me to lunch the following Tuesday. I agreed.

He was standing at the maître d' table, and as soon as he saw me walk in, he stepped forward, his hand extended, a big smile on his face.

"Hi Shary, I'm Patrick."

He was handsome, five foot eleven, with dark reddish-brown hair, sea-foam-green eyes, freckles, a crooked but inviting smile, and an athletic body. Dressed impeccably in a navy business suit and a striped red tie, Patrick seemed to be the consummate young Fortune 500 salesman. Polished. Charming. Self-assured. Ambitious. Take charge. I knew the type. I had worked with hundreds of salespeople over the years. I'd married one. He brushed my elbow as the hostess led us to our booth in the dark corner of the Chinese restaurant. I liked that he was chivalrous and took the lead. I felt cared for and excited already.

Over bites of chicken stir-fry, Patrick and I shared stories about our respective jobs, past relationships, travel, and sports. He locked his gaze on me. His playful eyes and mischievous grin were bait, beckoning me. Still I was guarded. My trust in men had eroded. Except for a pitiful blind date three months prior, this was my first date since my divorce almost two years ago.

But Patrick was funny, upbeat, and easy to talk to—just like it had been at the beginning with John. When we'd first started dating, John and I talked on the phone for hours. He was sensitive, caring, refreshingly connected to his feelings. Then that all changed. Now, listening to Patrick—who at just twenty-six, seven years younger than I was, sounded grounded, clear about who he was and what he wanted out of life—I was skeptical. Was he for real?

"You know yourself pretty well, don't you?" I asked, a little too antagonistically.

He smiled. "I've heard that before. One of the nuns I had in high school told me I was in touch with my feminine side," he said without a hint of embarrassment.

I was intrigued. I felt my neck relax. I leaned back and stretched my legs under the table. We sipped green tea as we meandered further into talk of career and travel.

"I'd love to move to the West Coast, to California, someday," I said. "San Diego is gorgeous. And NCR has a couple of manufacturing plants out there. So who knows?"

"That sounds wonderful," he said. "If you do move to the West Coast, I'd be interested in being a roommate." He looked directly at me, a seductive smile edging his lips.

"Oh. Uh. Okay," I mumbled, my posture tightening again. "I prefer living alone, but you never know."

"So, what exciting trips do you have coming up?" he asked, shifting his weight and draping his arm across the red velvet banquette.

"I'm headed to San Francisco next month to see my sister, and I have to go to New York to meet with the agency. And I'm thinking about a trip to Cape Cod in the fall. I've always wanted to go."

"Well, if we're still seeing each other then, maybe we can go together," he said.

For God's sake, it was our first date! My stomach gripped and my throat clenched with anxiety, the same way I'd felt when John hurried to get married, well before I was ready, the ink on his divorce barely dry. I'd prefer a slower dance. Still, I was flattered. Excited. The rush of being wanted felt so good! How exhilarating it was to feel attractive and desirable again. Patrick paid the check and escorted me to the parking garage.

"How about a movie Thursday night?" he said.

A movie on a weeknight? I didn't date during the week. I had to be at the office early in the morning.

And yet I heard the response tumble out of my mouth. "Sure, that would be great."

· ☙ ·

Insatiable

Back at the office that afternoon, I couldn't stop thinking about Patrick. My temporary stint on the hostile takeover team had concluded a week earlier; AT&T's acquisition of NCR was imminent. I was back in my old, mundane strategic marketing job, already plotting my next career move, dreaming about a six-month sabbatical. Two hours later, Patrick called to confirm our movie date for Thursday.

"It's going to be a beautiful evening tonight. Why don't we go for a walk?" he asked.

I had planned to go to the gym and meet my best friend, Kathy, afterward.

"That sounds wonderful. How would 6:30 work?" I said.

I gave him directions to my place with a buoyant "See you soon" just as he was saying the same.

"Jinx!" he said.

We laughed. How fun he is, I thought. God, how I needed to laugh and be lighthearted.

I left the office at 5:30, stopped at the wine store for a bottle of merlot and cheese and crackers, and headed home to call Kathy to apologize. I vacuumed, Windexed the guest bathroom, lit a wild-flower-scented candle, took a quick bubble bath, and dove into my closet for an appropriate second-date walk-in-the-park outfit. Sadly, my closet was stuffed with business suits and gym clothes and very little in between. I swept through each item hanger by hanger and flung a few sweaters and a pair of black chinos across the bed to study them for snags or lint. I threw on a black turtleneck and a fuchsia cardigan over the chinos. My heart was speeding. *I've got to calm down. I just met this man for the first time five hours ago, and he is coming over to my house in thirty minutes. Isn't this crazy? Is he as excited about me as I am about him? Oh my God, I've got to breathe.*

At 6:30 sharp, peering out my kitchen window, I saw him jog up the stone steps to the front door, looking at ease in a soft, brown leather jacket and khakis, with Ray-Bans dangling in his hand. God, he was sexy: baseball-toned body, just the right amount of freckles. After a long hibernation, my body was yawning awake, ravenous for touch and warmth. I'd not been affectionate with a man for more than two years. God, please help me be controlled and cautious. Let me take it slow, I prayed.

We took an hour walk in the Hills and Dales Park, adjacent to my home, strolling along the serene pathways as Patrick shared more about his family, college years, and playing football. Our conversation flowed effortlessly. I loved connecting with new people and was able to build a warm rapport quickly. I spent most of our walking time discovering more about Patrick, listening intently, and deferring questions about myself.

"You're so easy to talk to. I'm telling you things I haven't told anyone in years," Patrick said. "Thank you for listening."

I smiled. There was nothing I'd rather be doing in that moment than being with this fascinating man on a lovely spring evening. Pear and apple blossoms painted the monotone gray sky with gorgeous white, pink, and green strokes. Snowy white mounds of honeysuckle cascaded toward the sidewalks, embracing us.

"Isn't the honeysuckle intoxicating?" I said. He grabbed a branch of a voluptuous bush and pulled it to his nose, inhaling the sugary perfume.

"God, that's beautiful," he said. "I've never noticed these trees before."

Returning to my house hungry, we ordered sandwiches from a sub shop and picnicked in my living room. To ward off the early spring chill, I made hot chocolate doctored with Baileys Irish Cream for him and Amaretto for me topped with fluffy whipped cream and cinnamon. Mozart's piano concertos played softly in the background as we talked for hours about our careers, families, and past relationships. I looked at this secure and mature new man with anticipation, eager to learn more about him. Still, I was ill at ease. As much as I felt exhilarated, chomping at the bit for fresh love, I was reluctant.

"I don't want to taint any relationship with my muddied, messy past," I said. I was still aching from the crush of the divorce, and I knew I was vulnerable. "I'm still in transition, still finding my way. It's not fair to dump all of that on you."

"That's who you are and what you bring to a relationship," he said. "It's not a detriment. You can't think of it that way."

Already, he seemed so wise and understanding. His gentle, caring words were like lavender balm comforting me.

Patrick looked at me as if he were studying me.

"Your face looks tense," he said.

"Your pupils are so big," he had told me at lunch. "It shows that you're interested."

I was not used to such scrutiny. Although I was delighted by his attentiveness, I kept telling myself not to get involved with this guy. He was too young for me. Before John, I'd dated older men, much older in some cases. Worldly, sophisticated, financially comfortable, and someone I could respect and learn and grow with—that's what I wanted. I'd never been attracted to younger men. I shared this with Patrick.

"Well, it seems to me that your past image of the ideal mate hasn't been working," he said. "Maybe it's time to explore other options. Besides, look at it this way. A younger guy like me will be around a lot longer. Your old geezer might keel over."

He had a point. He seemed to be the kind of guy who had a ready response to any objection.

It was after midnight on a "school night," and I was fading. Patrick got up from the couch and wrapped the velvet coverlet around his waist, laughing and shaking his hips in a hula.

"Would you like to dance?" he asked.

"I'd love to. But maybe another time. I've got to get some sleep," I said.

I led him to my front door and reached out for a handshake to intercept our awkward first kiss, something I was nowhere near ready for. I felt a little smug being in control again. I had to slow things down.

"Well, goodnight, Miss Hauer." He smiled. "Are we still on for Thursday night? A movie or dinner or maybe watching a video at my place? Or are you sick of listening to me babble on all night?"

"Of course not. Let's get together."

The next day, less than twenty-four hours after meeting him, I was obsessed with Patrick, already consumed with waiting, wondering when his next call would come. My mind spun, speculating what he was thinking. I replayed and analyzed our conversations, coaching myself to reel in my emotions, play it cool, not appear too eager, put the brakes on my hungry heart. I remembered a friend's advice about transition relationships: just have fun, keep it light. Between business calls and meetings, my eye was glued to the phone and the red message light. Did he call? What is he thinking? Did I go too far, too fast in telling my friends that I met someone special? Did I chase him away with my defensiveness?

"What if I threw you on the couch and kissed you right now?" he asked me two nights later while we were enjoying carryout cheeseburgers in his apartment kitchen.

"Good luck trying," I said.

His face knotted into an exaggerated pout. "So, that's the way it's going to be, is it?" he asked half-jokingly, knowing full well it wasn't.

After dinner, he inched next to me on his bed as I flipped through his family photo album.

"Don't worry, I won't attack you," he said.

"Not a chance," I batted back.

"Wow, you're tough."

"Yeah, I know. I'm sorry. I guess I'm a bit defensive."

And frightened. And clueless. And desperate for yet avoiding your kisses. I was a jumbled mess. Patrick had been in my life for a mere three days and I could not get anchored. I struggled to make sense of my racing emotions, new hopes, old fears—men always hurt me—real urges, and painful memories, and they all sloshed around in a bucket of inner slop. Yet I was ecstatic thinking about my promising new romance. I was resurrected. Hope and hormones pulsed through my veins. Patrick was rescuing me, giving my life meaning and purpose again.

By the third date, I realized that Patrick had already etched his life plan, with marriage and children prominent in the blueprint. Each time we were together, he casually slipped an "If we got married . . . ," or "If we fall madly in love . . . ," or "If we have children . . . ," into our conversations.

"In seven years, you'll be forty," he said on one of our walks. "And you'll probably need to start having children no later than thirty-five, so you have two years to get this sabbatical thing out of the way."

Does he have me, us, already figured out? Why do I feel like I'm walking into a web? Can't we slow this down? One day, one week at a time? Don't talk and plan months in advance. Please.

61

Despite feeling anxious about Patrick's presumptuousness, my obsessiveness intensified. I thought about him constantly and fantasized about being with him every moment. I tortured myself waiting for his calls. When I didn't hear from him for thirty-six hours after our third date, my frenetic, sleep-deprived mind went haywire.

"I have a sick tearing in my gut," I wrote in my journal. "I haven't heard from him and all I do is wonder. I want to chop my head off or drink or do anything to stop this mindless torment, analyzing, questioning: Why hasn't he called? What in the world did I do? Did I chase him away?"

Through a torrent of tears, I desperately tried to get a grip. It was as if my right foot was pressed down on the gas pedal accelerating—"YES! YES! YES!" to Patrick—while my left foot was slamming on the brakes, imploring me not to express my feelings for the situation would only lead to heartbreak. My desire to deeply love someone clashed with the very real fear that if that actually happened, the result would be disastrous: another excruciating breakup.

Although I believed that Patrick should be the one to pursue me, by week two that rule had flown out the window. I couldn't wait to talk to and see him again, especially if a day or two had gone by. Especially if I imagined even the slightest bit of nonchalance in his voice on the phone. If he didn't ply me with compliments and innuendoes in every conversation, I got anxious and called him with an invite to stop over at my house after work so I could get my fix.

Over the next two weeks, we had a blast, dining out, playing puttputt golf, seeing movies, and walking in parks in my neighborhood. Although I was exhausted from weeks of late nights and sleep deprivation, I was flying with boundless energy. I was on a high with a drug that I told myself was too good to be true.

Unlike my ex-husband, whose life seemed to be divided into two pieces of pie—work and basketball—Patrick was multifaceted, enjoying his work, softball, racquetball, nature, being an extra in a movie filming downtown, taking acting classes, and learning how to draw. I was fascinated. I called him my Renaissance man. He was also a dreamer and a go-getter. He was interviewing for a promotion that could take him to Cincinnati or Atlanta, and many of our talks started to steer toward his career and how to handle escalating issues with his boss.

One Wednesday, I called him at the office to invite him to see the musical *Cats* on Saturday night at the Victoria Theatre downtown, where I was a season ticket holder. We talked briefly about our respective plans for the evening: he was headed to a concert in Cincinnati with a friend, and I had to be at a farewell party for one of my teammates.

"Why don't you stop over before you go?" I said.

"I'd love to," he said.

I left the office at four, fed up with the day, the week, my neck and back tense and achy. A half hour later, I held his hand and we walked up the winding staircase to my bedroom, where we lay clothed, side by side, on my antique cherrywood bed. His arms encircled me, and he kissed me lightly on my cheeks, forehead, and eyelids. "Butterfly kisses," he called them. I was captivated by his soft touch, his gentleness, as he patiently, slowly, teasingly avoided my lips. I wanted none of it. Rather all of it. Now. My body was greedy for his. I inched closer, nestling, nearly begging. What seemed like hours later, he slowly moved his lips to mine and tenderly kissed me.

"Why don't we run off to Rome, get married, and . . . ," he said.

I responded only by clutching his taut shoulders and nuzzling nearer to his chest. Finally, my body relaxed and I purred with contentment. I imagined staying right there, wrapped around him in our cozy hideaway, forever. Secluded from the demands of life. Just us. Just Patrick, fixing all of his attention on me. Me, schlubby me, with this Adonis in my bed, playing out my very own enchanting Cinderella fantasy. How had I gotten so lucky?

· ·

That Saturday night, he arrived at 5:30, and we enjoyed a quick glass of merlot before leaving for the theater. As he helped me with my coat and led me to the door, I took a deep breath—*God, he is handsome. So polished in his business suit*—as I fixated on his rear end. Once we were seated, I couldn't concentrate on the play with him so near. My body was zipping with electricity. I rested my head on his shoulder as he whispered in my ear and softly grazed my arm, my hand, my face, lightly kissing me. My arm tingled. How glorious it was to be the subject of so much affection. "Get a room!" I imagined those seated around us thinking.

After the show we returned to my place for a nightcap. I was in heaven, nestled in my living room with Patrick, relishing the scent of Amaretto-laced hot cocoa and Andrés Segovia's Spanish guitar playing in the background. On my way to the kitchen to refill our mugs, I changed the cassette tape to "You've Lost That Lovin' Feelin'."

"Oh, I can't believe it," he said. "The next song is 'Unchained Melody.' That's what I'm going to play at my wedding reception. Let's dance."

We embraced, drifting slowly across the living room floor. My usual awkward self, sure I'd step on his foot or bump into the coffee table, I tried to focus on the significance of the moment: our first dance. The first of many, I hoped. When the song ended, we sat down, and I resumed sipping my drink.

"Aren't you done with that hot chocolate yet?" he asked, smiling.

"No, I'm still savoring," I said, gripping the mug.

"I want a hug." He sat down beside me, took the mug from my hand, scooted it on the coffee table, and enveloped me in his arms. My strategy to play hard to get vanished in seconds as we necked on the couch for the next hour or so.

"Shall we retire to the boudoir?" I asked in my best French accent. He nodded. I scurried to the sitting room to insert a Kenny G cassette in the stereo, escorted him up the stairs, turned off the lights, and lit four small candles in my bedroom windows. We lay next to each other, kissing passionately, our clothes on, he gently covered his body with mine, our body heat rising, my desire to feel more of him surging as I rolled on top of him for a few moments.

"Shary, I want to please you so much, to give you pleasure," he whispered.

I sighed. My desire for Patrick unfurled. But I stopped. Pulled away. I wasn't ready to go all the way with Patrick. It was too soon. I had to protect myself. I knew that once I made love with him, my wanting, my need, my expectations would turbo thrust into a new galaxy, where my obsession knew no bounds. I already felt like a fool wanting to blurt out love messages to him. I was physically ready but emotionally unprepared. Given my history with men, I knew that I fell in love very easily, very quickly after having sex for the first time. Like many women, I became emotionally invested after making love. Only for me, once I surrendered to sex, I assumed a commitment was in the cards and I became full-bore, 24/7 man-obsessed. I was already crazy about Patrick.

Also at play, I'm sure, were several embedded beliefs I had about sex: my Catholic-school upbringing had taught me about Mary and the virtues of staying a virgin; my friend Laurie, whom I considered an expert in the relationship department, advised that I wait six months. That's when you know a man is serious, she said. The loudest voice of all was my mother's. A virgin when she married and the daughter of a floozy, she'd always warned me that men were after only one thing. Once they got it, they would flee unless you had a ring on your finger, she said. Mostly, I was convinced that putting off sex with a man would temporarily stem my deepest fear: being rejected and abandoned by someone I loved. I told myself that I needed to build a sense of trust and security with Patrick. I needed to know that he was committed first. I wanted a relationship that was sustainable, not throwaway. My driving compulsion, as a love addict, was to feel wanted by a devoted man who would give me perpetual romantic attention, a deep emotional attachment, and permanent safeness. It was not about the sex at all. Sex was lovely for the first six months. Then it became a duty. Sex addicts, on the other hand, are preoccupied with sexual intercourse, and it is often impersonal. Emotional attachment is typically not a factor.

"Only when you're ready," Patrick reassured me. "We'll take all the time you need." I was relieved that the pressure was off. He understood. We lay next to each other holding hands, sleeping on and off through the night.

At five o'clock the next morning, I went downstairs to turn the stereo off and take out my contacts and back up to try to sleep. Patrick was in a deep slumber. I could not relax my mind or body with him so near, so I tiptoed out of the bedroom to brush my teeth and touch up my makeup. I quietly emptied the dishwasher, made a pitcher of orange juice, and sat in the sunroom to glance at the newspaper, dizzy with sleeplessness. After he awoke at 11:00, we talked and snuggled until we realized it was almost 1:00 p.m. He had to be at a family baptism at 1:30. The race was on.

"Here we go again," I said. I hated to end our tryst in my nest prematurely. It seemed we were always in a rush, there was always something keeping us apart.

"There's nothing wrong with enjoying something until the very last moment," he said.

He brushed his teeth and splashed water through his hair. I poured him a glass of orange juice and stood in the kitchen humming as he walked in. He looked fresh and handsome, casually strolling in with a big "good morning" smile. I was bewitched. I'd entered dangerous territory. My desire for him was all-consuming; my controlled, rational self was on holiday. I thought about him all the time. Although I kept telling myself to be free-spirited, casual, nonchalant, and open to other relationships—to refrain from getting glued to him—it was too late. I was glued.

Two days later, I was sitting in the Pittsburgh airport at 6:00 a.m. eating popcorn and drinking a Diet Pepsi for breakfast, scanning *The New York Times* and *EuroTravel Magazine,* thinking and writing about Patrick. I was on my way to San Francisco for a week to visit my youngest sister, thankful for the chance to sleep, collect myself, and refocus. Yet all I could think about was calling him. Instead, I walked over to a candy and nut kiosk to buy a bag of banana chips. I was hungry. Still. After having dinner at 2:00 a.m., just four hours earlier, I laughed to myself, thinking about what a crazy night it had been.

We had pulled into my driveway at midnight after seeing a movie, only to find that we were locked out of the house. I had left my keys on the kitchen counter in a rush to make it to the movie on time. Unfortunately, there were no easy ways to enter my house. As rain started pouring, and as thunder and lightning cracked all around us, we took cover in Patrick's car and called a locksmith. An hour later, the lights from locksmith's truck flashed behind us, and we reluctantly got out of the car to greet him. We stood in the pelting, cold rain, barely covered by the dripping awning above my side door. Bud, with a flashlight in his mouth, quietly picked the lock. Patrick and I huddled close together behind him, our tongues roving inside each other's mouths.

"This doesn't seem to be working," Bud said. "I'm going to have to get my drill to take the lock apart." He ran off to his truck.

"My drill is ready," Patrick whispered in my ear. He pressed against me.

We eventually got back into the house where we downed a dinner of Diet Cokes, chips, and turkey sandwiches. Sadly, there would be no nookie this night. I had a flight to catch in just a couple of hours. But every inch of me ached to stay right there with Patrick, to continue where we had left off the other night. Reluctantly, we walked to my front door where we stood saying and kissing our good-byes for another hour. I couldn't let go.

Just as I feared, the small part of my brain that reason-checked was now unshackled. My emotions took on a life of their own, and my heart became even more demanding, more convinced that this was not a fling but something long term. Even though a new job and relocation for him were imminent, I marched on. After all, he'd asked me whether I'd move to Cincinnati or Cleveland or the Carolinas. I had to be part of his plan.

And yet my wise inner voice, normally mute when I was head over heels, did manage to utter doubt once or twice: Why did he insinuate that we were a couple with a long-term future so quickly? Why did he mention it every time we got together? Was he that certain about us?

Pleased yet fearful, I tried to tell myself not to take his innuendoes seriously. My heart and brain ping-ponged. Was this just a temporary thing or something permanent? I felt forced to classify the relationship, compelled to know exactly what it was, how he felt about me, us. Isn't this supposed to be spontaneous, frivolous, fun? But I was not letting it happen. I couldn't. I didn't want to feel out of control—not realizing I already was.

· ·

We got home late from a Cincinnati Reds game a few nights after I returned from San Francisco and settled into the living room for a nightcap. I turned the stereo on to play George Winston's soothing *Winter into Spring* piano melodies, made steaming hot cocoa, and surprised Patrick with a decadent chocolate cake I had made for his twenty-seventh birthday. Afterward, we wrapped our bodies around each other, partially clothed, kissing and caressing and getting dangerously close to intercourse. My body rubbing and grinding against his, I had my first orgasm in God knows how many years, and it was wonderful to feel so alive again.

After a few hours of sleep, I brought breakfast to bed: fresh strawberries, orange juice, leftover birthday cake on bright linens and flowery china, like a spring picnic in a Cotswolds Garden. We tasted and chatted and nested until four in the afternoon. To be wrapped around this man all day and night, just the two of us in our secret lair with not a care, was heaven.

"This looks like it's from a magazine spread or TV show," he said. "You are reopening my eyes to so many beautiful things."

I wanted to be with Patrick every moment. I couldn't keep my hands off him. Sleepless night after sleepless night, I surged with energy. I was high on love. Literally.

By the end of our first month together, Patrick's career talk dominated our conversations as he sought and I dispensed advice on his career, résumé, interviews, and wardrobe. Although I loved being needed, I began to resent his self-absorption and capitalizing our free time. He'd run rampant updating me on inconsequential details about his day, his career, his problems, his life.

One evening, weary from a trying week at the office, I wanted nothing more than to avoid work talk, to play and be silly with Patrick. Instead, he inventoried every grievance he had piled up with his boss over the past two years. Always the pleaser, I revved my natural caretaking role into high gear to spend the next two hours strategizing the pros and cons of resigning, and role-playing potential responses from his boss. "Is he another John?" I pondered in my journal. "Initially caring, concerned, sensitive, but a real asshole who cares only for himself and his own future?" I was angry, but I did not even think back then that I could insert myself into our talks. Worse, I feared the outcome if I did so. If I redirected my interest in him, would he lose interest in me? I continued to listen and fix. That's the role I had always played. That's all I knew.

Patrick started to not show up on time. He didn't call when he was going to be late; he cancelled a lunch or two at the last minute. I was upset, feeling taken advantage of but didn't say so. I wanted only to please, not cause a ruckus. I had no idea of boundaries—what healthy, acceptable behavior was supposed to be in a new relationship. I accepted all responsibility and prayed that I'd be more understanding, forgiving, and patient, even when Patrick was in the wrong.

• •

After holding off on making love with Patrick for almost two months, I finally relented. It was late afternoon on an unseasonably warm Saturday, the open windows inviting only the faintest breeze. The soft fragrance of dainty lilies of the valley in a crystal vase on the windowsill wafted through the room. We undressed and I awkwardly slid into bed, covering my body with the cotton sheet while he stood at the foot of the bed naked, smiling, as if on display. Patrick played the maestro, conducting a perfectly choreographed performance of velvety touch and kisses. He held me with care, moving his body in concert with mine, tenderly looking into my eyes, entering me effortlessly as if it were all prearranged. I was delirious, resuscitated by a man who adored me.

"My God, you are amazing. You can go on and on and on," I said, still catching my breath, the sheet crumpled across our bodies.

"I know my product," he said, smirking.

Two weeks later, after we had oral sex for the first time, I didn't hear from Patrick for days afterward. During the previous few weeks he had been "busy" more often—less time for us, late for our dates without an explanation, canceling plans. I tried to empathize: during that brief time frame, he had had a disagreement with his boss that had cost him his job, he had started a new job, and, tragically, his high school girlfriend had been killed in an auto accident in Pennsylvania. He was understandably distraught and remote. Yet because the turnaround in him was so abrupt, I was anxious, panicky, unable to sleep, and I couldn't help but rack my brain for explanations. My fear of cold, stark abandonment seeped in like a slow-drip chemo.

"I'm in a transition. I'm confused," Patrick said in a phone call I initiated a week later. His voice was flat, void of his typical exuberant energy and flirty quips. "I think it's best if I don't pursue a relationship—that we're not intimate right now. We'll get together when you get back."

I was leaving on a trip to Spain with my sister in three days. I didn't want to go. I wanted to be with him. To make us better again. Bring back his gentle, sexy voice and hard body to hold.

I didn't hear from him again. No explanation. No, here's why I pursued you like a wild leopard and dropped you like a stinky skunk. Nothing. A cold, barren, heartless kick to the curb.

When I returned from Spain, I was still reeling. Anxious. Still fixated on Patrick. I hated being alone. Again. Lost and bereft without the rapturous fuel of a man's passion. Although I knew I had to focus on reinvigorating myself and getting my career on a happier track, emptiness and anger drained me. I thrashed around in thoughts of what could have been rather than what needed to be. My friends attempted to comfort me. Wise Laurie and her husband, Joe, who had joined Patrick and me for happy hour a few times, validated what I refused to see: Patrick was self-centered.

"He certainly needed an inordinate amount of attention," Laurie said. And who better to give it to him than me, an expert in catering to others' egos.

"He wasn't ready for a serious relationship," Joe said.

Now they tell me! And my best friend, Kathy, counseled me with the same words I had shared with her many times: let this time, this free time, be a time for you to focus your energy on you.

But I wasn't able to move on like other women seemed to do. My wounds were too deep. Accustomed to heartbreak and suffering, I replayed memories and spun tales of what could have been. I still hoped he'd appear at my doorstep or call or send a Christmas card or be sitting behind me in church or driving next to me on the highway. I told myself it was just a three-month fling, a transition relationship, a pleasant diversion, nothing more. Move on. Yet the louder part of me imagined he was the love of my life. At the same time, I was angry. Seething. Another man coldly heaving me aside. With no explanation. Cowardice.

The next month, when I took a long-weekend trip to Lake Erie with my mom and dad and four- and six-year-old nieces, the left side of my face fell. I didn't know anything was wrong until my mom screeched, "Oh my God, you're having a stroke!"

I looked in the mirror. The entire left side of my face had dropped several inches. My left eye was nearly shut, and my lips on that side were downturned into a sliding frown that caused a mumbled lisp. That afternoon, back home in Dayton in the emergency room, I was diagnosed with Bell's palsy. Who gets Bell's palsy at thirty-three? Those who are heartbroken and drowning in self-induced anguish, fueled by a shot of anger, apparently. Many years later, I discovered that Bell's palsy is caused by an extreme attempt to control anger, an inability to express feelings, according to mind/body healer Louise Hay.

Five months after our breakup, I was still consumed and comforted by memories of us. I was convinced that I would never find someone as perfect as Patrick—someone I had so much in common with, who shared so many of my interests and feelings, who had the same enthusiasm for the simple things in life that I did. I realized years later that it wasn't so much that I missed him; it was losing my dream of him. How could I possibly let go of something I thought I'd never have again? I'll never have love like this again. That's the lie I told myself.

After going through the emotional wringer of a traumatic breakup and divorce, we may not realize how romantically vulnerable we are. The urgent desire to find someone new can cloud good judgment. And in love addiction, as in any addiction, there is typically a lack of sound judgment. Ignoring the red flags and the voice that says, "slow down," we can get sucked in again by the thrill and excitement of seductive words and touch and drama and conflict—the stuff many of us have become conditioned to expect.

5

The Good Guy

In 1992, a year after my breakup with Patrick, I was in a new role at NCR—now officially called AT&T Global Information Solutions. As the director of marketing communications for the Personal Computing Division, I was excited about abandoning the stuffy corporate position that I had slogged in for two years, creating presentations about esoteric global technology strategies. The personal computing business was in its heyday in the early '90s: Apple had just introduced the world's first PDA—personal digital assistant—and credit-card-sized memory storage devices were all the rage. My team and I touted innovations like the AT&T Safari laptop, the world's first personal computer with a built-in modem and networking, to the international computer press, *The Wall Street Journal* and *The New York Times*.

One afternoon, a couple of months into my new job, a blond, preppy-looking guy with an Opie smile appeared at my office door to deliver a package from a colleague.

"Hi, I'm Doug," he said. "I'm an intern working for Joy in the Latin America group. Here's the document you requested."

"Thank you," I said. I had a meeting in five minutes and needed to prepare. I picked up a report on my desk and started to read it. Doug stood outside my office, still grinning at me as if he wanted to talk more. God, he looked so young and boyish. Like a party boy. Certainly not the suit-and-tie corporate type I was attracted to.

"Thanks again. I'll see you soon," I said.

Two weeks later, on a steamy pre–Labor Day evening, my coworker and friend Joy and I and several of her teammates, including Doug, rented a ten-passenger van and drove to see Elton John at Riverbend, a popular outdoor concert venue on the banks of the Ohio River in Cincinnati. Joy and I had reserved seats in the pavilion, and despite the oppressive heat, we sang and danced to "Rocket Man" and "The Bitch Is Back" like teenage groupies.

At intermission, I walked outside to buy a bottle of water and on my way back to our seats, I saw Doug drinking an icy soda, people watching. After raving about Elton's first set and complaining about the weather and crowds, we quickly diverted to my favorite topic, traveling. I had been in San Francisco over the Fourth of July weekend, and I was so enthralled with the weather and fabulous California cuisine. He'd just returned from Andros Island in the Bahamas, a spot I'd always wanted to visit.

"It's quiet and peaceful—Zen-like," he said. "And the water is so clear. The fishing is fantastic. I stayed at the Green Turtle Inn on the outskirts of the island, right on the Caribbean. I've got a brochure at home that I can bring in for you if you'd like."

"That would be great," I said. "Thank you."

As Doug worked in the Latin America group, I asked him if he spoke Spanish or had ever been to South America.

"Not yet," he said.

"I love everything Latin," I said. "What little I know of it growing up in southern Ohio."

I do not recall all that our first conversation entailed, but I do remember thinking, *there's something interesting about this guy.* He was deeper, more intriguing than I had judged him to be earlier. Even though he was younger than I was, he seemed to have a wise and mature air about him, and I sensed a spiritual quality. Perhaps behind that happy, big-teeth-grinning, towheaded frat-boy persona was potentially a man of substance.

The next week I returned to my office from lunch and saw a long-stemmed red rose and a handwritten note on my desk. I wasn't sure what the message said—it was written in Spanish—except for the last line asking me to dinner Saturday night. It was signed by Pepe Armando. I didn't know a Pepe Armando. Could he be Doug's alter ego? I knew he didn't speak or write Spanish, so he must have convinced a colleague to collaborate. Of course I accepted.

We had dinner at El Meson, an authentic slice of South America plunked down next to I-75 in Dayton. Sitting outside on the brick patio, bowers of cherry red and lilac bougainvillea draping above, sipping a lusty Carménère, I felt as if we were dining in an ancient courtyard in sultry Buenos Aires. Our conversation flowed with ease. I liked that Doug asked me questions about my life, my dreams, and listened with care. He didn't talk too much about himself. He wasn't trying to impress and woo me. John and Patrick had come on too strong from the get-go with premature innuendos of a future together. Although their pushiness made me feel anxious and apprehensive, I was instantly seduced by their daring and dash. Confidence was something I had tasted only once or twice in my life. As if symbiotic, I needed to attach myself to a fearless and commanding man. But Doug was different—calm, humble, and self-assured in a subtle, knowing way. When he smiled at me across the table with his warm and sincere blue eyes, it seemed he understood the deepest part of me already. I agreed to have dinner with him the following Saturday.

· ·

Three weeks later, on a Saturday afternoon, we were standing outside The Horseshoe, the famous Ohio State stadium in Columbus. Doug had scored coveted tickets for a home football game and planned every detail of the day, making sure we had plenty of time to enjoy the tailgating craziness before the game. It was a cold, cloudy, and windy October day and Doug came prepared. We sat huddled together in heavy coats and gloves, our legs and knees covered by warm stadium blankets he had packed, as we sipped his homemade hot toddies from a steaming Thermos. Even our rear ends were protected from the cold steel bleachers with the soft stadium cushions he had brought. He had thought of everything. I didn't need to do a thing. How wonderful!

Within a month, we were seeing each other every weekend. In the beginning, I resisted moving into a serious relationship with Doug. Or tried to. I called it a transition relationship. Transitioning from what to what, I did not know. But it was comforting to think of it that way. Doug was finishing his MBA and was a few months from graduation.

I told myself he was too young—twenty-six, nine years younger than I was—and that I wasn't magnetized to him like I was to alpha males like John and Patrick. Yet I had been pummeled attempting repeatedly to win and keep the love of those rejecting men. Perhaps my unconscious self was telling me it was time for a dramatic change, that I needed a kinder, gentler relationship with a man who would nurture and care for me, not just himself.

Underneath all of my "Should I proceed with Doug?, Should I back out?" questioning, I realize now that the decision had already been made. I'd never stand a chance trying to override the trifecta of constants that unconsciously governed my life: (1) I was always famished for a man's attention, (2) I needed to feel lovable again, and (3) I desperately feared feeling alone and empty without a man. I wasn't aware back then of how much I needed a fix, how dependent and starving I was for the exhilarating, all-consuming rush of being wanted by a man. And, right here in front of me, a smiling, lovable admirer was ready to give me his heart. I surrendered, allowing myself to fall into a relationship with a nice guy I really wasn't enamored with.

It didn't take long before I learned that Doug was attracted to me in part for my maturity and business sense. "You are the smartest businessperson I've ever met," he said one evening. Rather than being flattered, I thought *how naive*. Doug was just starting his career. I had fifteen years of corporate experience on him. I must have seemed worldlier and more accomplished. Certainly I knew I was light-years ahead of him in earning power. Although I was troubled by the discrepancies—I wanted a man who was, at a minimum, on par with me professionally and financially—I brushed my disappointment aside and focused instead on what I thought was more important: Doug's kindness and generosity.

Three months from getting his MBA, Doug was trying to figure out where to direct his job search and sought my counsel about the best companies to focus on. Soon I was dispensing advice on his résumé, wardrobe, and interviewing skills. Before I knew it, I was in the middle of another rehab project, reverting to my instinctual pattern of mothering and caretaking. This time, my subject was an eager underling.

Doug and I became intimate after a month and half of seeing each other. In my bed on a chilly Sunday morning, wrapped in a cozy down comforter, he hugged me tight and looked at me with such intensity.

"I love you," he said.

I was stunned. I looked into his eyes and remained silent. My stomach gripped with anxiety. It was way too soon to reciprocate. I didn't feel it. I felt horrible, like I was letting him down, inadequate for not being able to return his affection.

Looking back, it seems I had always had trouble distinguishing between a potential friend and a potential lover. With Doug, I was pretty certain, even at the beginning, that my heart did not envision him as "the one." The rational, knowing part of me, the part that I rarely gave a voice to, saw him as a comfortable companion—an amazingly dependable, loving, always-happy companion. But my addict self, the unaware part of me that craved attention no matter the source, settled and got involved with the wrong person for the wrong reasons to avoid the anguish of feeling alone.

· ·

In March 1993, Doug landed a terrific sales job with Johnson & Johnson calling on physicians in Cincinnati and northern Kentucky. He moved to an apartment in a growing suburb of Cincinnati, forty minutes south of my work and home. Our weekend-only relationship was easy and fun. Doug and I genuinely liked being with each other and loved planning our next get-together. We had a phone date every night at 9:00 p.m. during the week to talk, catch up on the day, and plan weekend adventures such as hiking in the local preserves, antiquing, and getting together with friends.

I don't remember when I started to wrest control of our relationship. It was very gradual; neither of us noticed. After six months or so, when I stopped feeling the rush from our new coupling my need to control stepped in. It began innocently. He asked me for my help and I gave it to him. Doug was laid back and agreeable, so it was easy for me to start making the decisions on where we'd go for dinner, what trips we would take, how we'd spend our weekends. Add in my unofficial role as his career coach and the balance of power in our relationship had definitely shifted from balanced to Shary is running the show. But beyond managing, I became more bossy, nagging, and bitchy. "God, you eat like a truck driver," I snapped when I saw him holding a dinner roll in his left hand while eating with his right. When I reviewed one of his business reports and it was riddled with grammatical errors, I admonished him like an evil schoolteacher. How did I go from being a warm, engaged lover for the first six months to a cold, critical mother? Typically, Doug didn't respond to my criticisms. If he did, he'd make light of it, which, in retrospect, gave me a green light to continue getting away with my belittling behavior.

What is clear to me now, two decades later, is that many of us love addicts who experienced little security in our childhood, have a desperate need to control our men and our relationships. Our goal is maintain the illusion of control so we can keep focusing on *him* in order to not feel a thing inside. We mask our efforts to control people and situations as being helpful, says author of the seminal book *Women Who Love Too Much* Robin Norwood.

Knowing what I know now, that real intimacy starts to develop at the six-months-or-so stage, I realize that that's when my unconscious red flags went up with Doug. My internal dialogue went something like this: "Danger, danger. I am getting attached to this person. What happens when I get attached? In the case of my parents, they ignore me and move on to another child. In the case of John and Patrick, they run. They abandon me." Deeply ingrained in my psyche was the message that people always hurt me, no matter how loving they appear. To protect myself from what I was certain was going to be painful, I unconsciously activated my trusty defense systems—being overly controlling and micromanaging. I feared intimacy. And the more afraid I was, the more controlling I became.

I know now that I was, in love-addiction terms, a "switch-hitter" with Doug. I had served as the passive pleaser with dominant, seductive, and self-absorbed John and Patrick. But with easygoing Doug, I reversed roles to become more of a narcissistic love addict—the taker and controller—and Doug served as a codependent—the pleaser. Switch-hitting among love addicts is not uncommon and is usually unconscious. In my case, I was absolutely unaware of my switching behavior.

Like a puppy, endlessly devoted and loving Doug was always there for me. I could trust and count on him. But I realize now that I was bored from the get-go. I wasn't accustomed to calm and peace in a relationship. I was never interested in the quiet, stable "good guys" like Doug—the type of man I could rely on, the ones who would really love me. I thrived on (a.k.a. was addicted to) and suffered from uncertainty and drama. I didn't have the pounding-in-the-heart feeling with Doug, the "I can't wait to see you," the "I don't want you to leave" feelings that I associated with true love. *Maybe this is what true love is supposed to feel like,* I thought. *Maybe this is the healthier, less needy, more mature version of love I've been wanting. Maybe real love is not meant to be turbulent.*

Some of us are afraid of intimacy and don't even know it. In fact, we would insist it's exactly the thing we most want. But for many who suffer from low self-esteem and loving too much, as Norwood describes, we "are not attracted to men who are kind, stable, reliable, and interested in us, the ones who want to be intimate and give us their heart. We find such 'nice' men boring." If we don't feel very good about ourselves, how can we handle a nice guy who treats us so well?

Despite my misgivings, I couldn't shake my need for Doug's companionship, and a year passed before I knew it. By our second year together, we had settled into our routine like an old married couple—an old married couple that saw each other on weekends. We had dinner at our favorite Vietnamese restaurant and a cheap movie on Friday night. Saturdays we worked around my house, raking piles of leaves deposited by the dozens of old oaks and maples, tending to the fruit trees, or playing Monopoly or Aggravation with my nieces and nephew. Sundays were relaxation days—except when it was golf season, when Doug religiously hit the links for eighteen holes—and I loved our easy, unscheduled brunches together, reading the newspaper, walking in neighborhood parks, and tending to my yard and home.

Unlike John, who had had a distant relationship with my family, Doug loved my family, and they loved him. He fit right in, and it was easy and comfortable to include Doug in our family get-togethers. Even my mom, who was standoffish, hyper-opinionated, and critical, liked Doug. "Gosh, he's cute," she whispered to me in my kitchen that first Easter, when I introduced him to my family. And he accepted her, even laughed at her surliness. One evening, seated next to my parents at a formal charity event, my mom and Doug got into a friendly debate about local politics. When she blurted, "Don't give me any of your shit, Doug," I almost doubled over in embarrassment.

I looked across the table to the other guests. Had they heard her? Doug just laughed. "Oh, Norma."

As an only child, Doug loved the holiday chaos of my large, noisy, bickering clan of brothers and sisters and their kids. He joined my brothers on the golf course and basketball court, energized by male trash-talking and camaraderie. He had endless patience when we occasionally babysat my four- and five-year-old nieces and had elaborate pretend tea parties. Doug was part of our family, a fact that, despite my earlier ambivalence about our relationship, further entrenched us.

· ·

I had been in the PC marketing job and the relationship with Doug for two years and I was at an all-time low. What had been building for several years, but I was only able to admit in recent months, was that I was not a good fit for large corporate cultures. I despised the fact that self-serving egos, gamesmanship, and constant machinations were prerequisites for success. I didn't understand the games, couldn't play them, and didn't want to. I felt trapped in a soulless cocoon. On and off for years, I tried to identify a new career path, to no avail. I knew I had the makeup of an entrepreneur. I needed to call my own shots, have the freedom to do the kind of work I wanted to do with terrific passionate people, and exercise creative muscles that seemed to have atrophied. I wanted to start my own business, but could not get focused. I had a zillion ideas—from specialty-food marketing to travel consultant to floral designer to working on movie productions—zipping in and out of my brain. I hired a renowned life design specialist in Miami and a career counseling firm in New York to help me get clear on my direction. But, I continued to stew and suffer. And I was feeling snippy, with low energy, when I was with Doug, and I didn't know why. I steadily grew unhappier and blasé about us. I disengaged. I had to force myself to kiss him. I avoided lovemaking as much as possible. I nitpicked him about his apartment, his weight, his driving. Everything was a source of complaint.

I felt dissociated from work, unconnected to everyone and everything. I had a conversation with my good friend Sheila, and it felt forced, full of effort. I went to happy hour on a Friday night with my colleague Alicia and the gang and I couldn't wait to get home. I talked with my mom and it was like talking to a wall. There was no connection. I felt hollow.

I had always suffered from bad PMS, but in the previous few years, the symptoms had been far worse. This was not PMS. Night after night of no sleep, no energy, constant hunger and thirst. My memory was foggier and foggier. My hair was falling out. I had anxiety attacks and zero desire for sex. Worse, I was getting more quick to anger, sometimes going straight to rage, and I seemed to erupt at the slightest provocation.

I made an appointment with Dr. Susan, the psychologist I started seeing after my divorce from John. Dr. Susan was a beacon of sensibility. She always talked practically, not clinically.

"You have chronic biological depression, likely since childhood," she said. "It's getting more pervasive—worse." The anger I had felt as a little girl had been bottled up for more than thirty years, she said. It propelled me to keep going. But now the lid was finally popping off my internal pressure cooker. The emotional blockages were now too deep to ignore. That was the first time I had heard or thought about the anger and sadness I had had as a little girl. I believed her—it all made sense—but I couldn't feel what she was talking about. Dr. Susan sent me to two of her colleagues: a psychiatrist, who immediately put me on an antidepressant, and an art therapist, who looked at my self-portrait, with my hair unattached to my oversized head, and instantly diagnosed me as disconnected. Disconnected from my feelings. Disconnected from life. That pretty much summed up how I felt.

The antidepressant wasn't the elixir I was hoping for, although it did help a little to modulate and even out the deep lows and emptiness I felt every day. Meanwhile, my work with Dr. Susan focused on getting me to feel the little-girl anger and sadness she said I had repressed. I penned unsent letters to my mom and dad, wrote essays about my life as a nine-year-old and a thirteen-year-old, went shopping in a toy store to recapture playfulness, and attempted to evoke the warmth and nurturing of my now-deceased grandmother. But as hard as I tried to feel the feelings, I could access only a handful of childhood memories. I was dissociated from my little-girl self. I wasn't sure I was making any progress at all.

By my third year with Doug, I was constantly wringing in guilt and remorse for being so unloving and disrespectful. I pulled away from him even further, and as I did, he demanded more. Never strongly or with anger, simply a firm expression that he needed more connection with me, more intimacy.

"It is so difficult," Doug said one night, looking at me with such earnestness and sadness. "You simply cannot accept the love that I want to give."

Our sexual contact dwindled to less than once a month. I was selfishly depriving Doug and myself of the intimacy we both needed. Denying myself pleasure was easy, automatic for me. I was used to neglecting my needs. But what I didn't realize, living in my myopic, egotistical world, was that by neglecting Doug's sexual needs, I was not valuing, honoring, and reassuring him as a man. The more pressure I felt to please Doug, the more I knew I was letting him down, the more disappointed in myself I became. *I can never stack up, be as kind and as unconditionally loving as he is,* I thought. Because I'd invested such superhuman qualities in Doug, I know now, I couldn't possibly accept any pleasure or love from him.

Although I diligently completed Dr. Susan's assignments, journaled, prayed relentlessly about being a nicer person, and gobbled *A Return to Love, The Road Less Traveled,* and other spiritually nourishing books, I continued to be critical of Doug and myself. I knew that my need to feel more secure, stronger, better, superior was wrong. I implored myself to STOP! But I couldn't. And didn't. I could not understand why I continued to destroy a relationship that was the best I'd ever had or wanted. I coached myself repeatedly to be more giving with Doug, to open my heart more. But I was stuck in the pattern of an abuser. Abuse, remorse. Abuse, remorse. Although I didn't call it that at the time.

Throughout it all, Doug was a constant, a rock, patiently supporting me, waiting for me to shed my demons, giving me plenty of room.

Doug was the first person in my life to help me realize how unloving I was to myself. He saw that I was attractive and compassionate and loving and competent, but I was blind to those things. His compliments fell on deaf ears. I brushed off his frequent appreciations. "I can feel so much love inside of you. What in the world are you saving it for?" he said. I had no clue. I didn't realize then that self-appreciation was something I needed to cultivate rather than depending upon a man to make me feel good. Doug didn't tolerate my constant self-flagellation either. When he heard me criticize myself, he'd stop me. Or try to. "My hope is for you to someday recognize how much love and beautiful karma you have to offer everyone around you," he wrote in one of his anniversary cards.

Despite achieving what had been my primary aim in life, winning the love of a man, the love that had been long withheld by my parents and other men, now that I had finally won the big prize, I didn't know what to do with it. Finally someone genuinely wanted to be close to me, and I couldn't handle it. I didn't recognize back then what I came to know thanks to relationship expert Harville Hendrix: parental rejection typically leads to self-rejection, which leads to an inability to receive love, which translates to an inability to give love. Knowing there were reasons for my destructive behaviors didn't excuse them, but it helped me become more understanding and compassionate with myself. And the truth about love addiction, now that I understand it a little more, is that it is not about real love at all. My illusion of love is what I was addicted to. I fed off my fantasies of romance, my idealized notions of intimacy, my outsize expectations of true love—they were what fueled me. But when I received the real deal—Doug's offer of his whole heart—I did everything I could to avoid and reject it.

My habit of chewing certain foods and not swallowing them, a habit I started in high school, escalated with Doug. I had always been twenty or thirty pounds overweight. I'd always had an uncontrollable craving for sugar, particularly cookies and pastries. I swallowed most food, but I spit out chewed doughnuts and snack cakes, which seemed like an innocent way to enjoy the foods I wanted without gaining more weight. On the one hand, it seemed harmless. I didn't vomit or purge.

I just spit the food out. In my mind it was nothing more than a dieting technique. On the other hand, I knew it was something shameful, because I had kept this secret to myself for almost thirty years.

As soon as Doug would pull out of my driveway on Monday mornings, after our weekends together, I'd hightail it to the Twinkie store—the Hostess outlet on the edge of downtown—to load up on breakfast rolls and cupcakes. Boxes of them. I'd shove them in one after another, the cinnamon iced rolls slathered in a coating of soft butter, then spit them out. In the same way, I ingested Doug's love like a thirsty vampire but was unable to receive it in my heart—and unable to reciprocate it. Instead I Novocain-ed the anxious pressure that gripped my throat and gut every weekend we were together. I could never be as kind, as giving, as unconditionally loving as he was. I binged on sweets to cram out the dark cavern of inadequacy. My addict self convinced me that I didn't need the intimacy that Doug offered. Instead I made love with baked goods.

I later found out, when I finally broke down and called an eating-disorder coach, that my habit is called oral expulsion. I learned that my lifetime habit was not innocent at all but destructive. I had an eating disorder. I was always alone when I did this, and it was always in secret. I saw a similar pattern with my mother: she'd rarely sit down to have meals with the family. Rather, she'd go off to her bedroom with a plate of food, hiding from the world.

As I learned much later, addiction feeds addiction. It's not uncommon for a love addict—or any addict—to have multiple addictions. For many alcoholics, an addiction to coffee and cigarettes goes hand in hand. A striking number of food addicts who have gastric bypass surgery turn to alcohol and/or drugs as substitutes. I happened to exchange Ding Dongs and Little Debbies for the love that I was addicted to but couldn't give or receive.

We soldiered on into a fifth year, the relationship slowly suffocating. I was even more detached; Doug was even more frustrated and vocal in expressing his unrequited needs. In less than one minute after walking into his apartment one Saturday afternoon, I attacked his attire—he wore an ancient and dirty oversized T-shirt, his eating habits—a box of Frosted Flakes sat on the counter, and after inspecting the new sofa and chair, his complete lack of decorating style.

"Stop. It. Now!" he yelled. "You pick constantly. You criticize and moan and control everything. I'm tired of it. Really tired of it." He had been patient and understanding, waiting to see improvement in my behavior for the previous four years, in vain. I felt more inadequate. Over and over again, I flogged myself for not being an adult and treating him with respect. I hated myself for not living up to his love. The subject of breaking up came up more frequently now, at least once a week, but neither of us walked away. When I thought about breaking up, the intense doom of losing my most ardent supporter and the dread of being alone devoured me. I could not let go. I could not be alone.

Because I couldn't see my way through the nasty hair ball of this complex relationship, I sought insight from a psychic, Debbie, for direction. "You both are very passionate," she told me when I asked her about Doug. "You are both very committed, both very spiritual. You have an energetic resonance—the energy waves between you two are really great. You are soul mirrors."

I took this as a sign. We're supposed to be together. I had a twinge of hope, then doubt. Second thoughts. Always second-guessing myself. *What's wrong with me? This guy is great.* Everyone loved Doug. Again, I'd remind myself that I would never find another man as loving, generous, and kind as Doug. He was the love of all loves. I'd berate myself for being unable to return his unconditional love. I sat in hours and hours of therapy, desperate to rehabilitate myself. This tug of war— this plodding, agonizing process—went on for almost six years. Of course, I often wondered why Doug continued to stay with me when I'd done all I could to chase him away.

"What you need is a real asshole," he said after one of my tirades. I'd already done that. More than once. No, I hadn't been better off. Only years later did I speculate about the possible depths of Doug's wounded self-esteem. Why else would he put up with my emotionally torturous behaviors? I didn't have enough insight back then to realize we were locked into what spiritual teacher Marianne Williamson refers to as the "push and pull of codependent neuroses." Looking back, it seems so easy now. *Just be kind and caring, Shary. It's not that difficult.*

But it was. To paraphrase Williamson: We don't think about being kind and caring; we think about how we can keep the man. We don't think about his fears and his problems; we think of our own and how we can get him to solve them. We don't think about him period. So true. So sad.

On a Sunday night in late September 1998, depleted by my inability to love him the way he loved me, exhausted from our endless pushing and pulling, we ended our six-year relationship. It wasn't planned. It just happened. I can't remember what provoked the tipping point, but there were tears and I ordered him to pack up his clothes and leave. It was that simple. We didn't say another word to each other that night. Ten days later, Doug stopped by my house to pick up the remainder of his belongings. He was taking the breakup harder than I was. He looked at me with his loving eyes, pleading for answers. I felt awful for hurting someone I loved so much. I wanted to make his pain go away. I found myself consoling him. Comfort Doug. Fix his pain. I was always fixing.

6
The Wreck Years

My father had a superhuman capacity for work, toiling in the family business to clothe, feed, and school six children. To fund our eventual college tuitions and cars, he launched another company in the 1970s, which put him on the road traveling to hi-fi dealers throughout Ohio, Kentucky, Indiana, and Tennessee every week. When Dad was home, he seemed emotionally vacant, unexpressive. At the time, I thought it was because he always had too much to do at home. Something needed fixing, the lawn had to be mowed, or one of my brothers had to go to peewee football practice or an Indian Guides meeting. I don't remember hugs or kisses or Dad asking me how school was going. Never a "How are you feeling?" or a "Tell me what's happening in your world" from either parent. Nor did I seek it. Their attention was elsewhere, often on one of my brothers, who wrestled, knocking furniture over and smashing holes in my mother's fine oil paintings.

Not surprisingly, I didn't know how men were supposed to behave. The Dick and Jane books I read in school depicted the man of the family as the patriarch, the stern but loving role model, the one the kids went to for permission to go to the store or play ball outside. I saw Jim, the father on *Father Knows Best,* as the dispenser of sage advice whenever one of his three children had a dilemma. And when Bud or one of the other kids got in trouble at school, their housewife mother, Margaret, always in a pretty dress and baking delicious after-school cookies, gently guided the child on how to approach fear-mongering

Dad, who would surely dole out a devastating punishment. But my dad was quiet and mostly passive. He rarely yelled and never issued punishment. If he did, my brothers ignored him. We obeyed and feared my mother, who rarely wore a dress and never baked cookies. Like all girls longing to be "daddy's girl," I wanted to be cherished and treasured by my father. I was desperate to recapture the tenderness, the bond I felt when he fixed his big, warm, brown eyes on mine as he fed me breakfast every morning when I was a baby. But, as with other girls whose fathers were emotionally distant, too busy working, or absent from the home, I didn't feel cherished. My self-assuredness was severely underdeveloped.

Feeling increasingly defective and alone, I turned inward to create new sources of love and attention. I studied television shows and looked in my mom's *McCall's* magazine and *Ladies' Home Journal* for pictures of happy and loving families. From time to time, I was comforted. But, mostly, seeing what I assumed was ideal love only intensified my yearning. Any little bit of male attention I got I inflated. When our neighbor Jill's dad took her and three of us ten-year-old girls on a weekend trip to the family's rustic cabin in southern Ohio, I was overjoyed when he asked me to sit in the front seat of the tractor, next to him, not in the back with the others. From that innocent gesture, I leaped to imagining him thinking I was more mature than his daughter, who couldn't stop whining about how cold it was. I hoped he had appreciated me helping him carry the lanterns and blankets to the tractor. I wanted him to see that I was special. And two years later, when handsome Mr. Bart, my science teacher, wrote "A" and "good job" on the cover of my photosynthesis report, I developed a little crush. I conjured scenarios in which he would compliment me for my science savvy and dole out extra attention to spur my learning. It was at this point—preadolescence—that I began to exaggerate the significance and intent of the slightest attention men showed me. I had no inkling then of how deeply I craved feeling valued by men. Little did I know that I would be consumed with trying to fill this void for the next four decades.

Along the way, I started to soothe my hunger by envisioning being rescued by a majestic king who adored me and was endlessly devoted to me. This little-girl fantasy, fueled by longing and melancholy, wasn't just an innocent ten-year-old's passing dream—it governed my entire adult life as my addiction to romance and love played out episode after episode. In each of my relationships, I was unable to see who the man really was. Instead I saw the rescuer image I had created in childhood. Even into my forties and early fifties, after years of counseling and healing, I was still stuck in my ten-year-old head and heart, continuing to see men as I wanted them to be, not as they were. It astonished me how grown-up and accomplished I was in all other parts of my life but how deluded and adolescent I was in my love life. I was a successful career woman on the rise. No one knew I was a highly functioning love addict.

At Incarnation School, most of the girls in my seventh-grade class were slim, with long, blond, straight hair. They wore jeans and makeup and flirted with boys. With a nest of frizzy curls, I was fat, zitty, and nearsighted. I wore easy-to-launder Danskin knit ensembles and special-order, size-E Buster Browns. Kathy, Stephanie, and especially Ann talked about boys and the stuff they did with them over the weekend, and I'd listen as if I were hearing Japanese for the first time. Being with a boy was that foreign to me. The only boy I'd ever been even remotely interested in was Bill, and I wasn't even sure why. Bill was cute and had short, dark, curly hair like mine, and he may have mumbled a "hi" or even managed what I interpreted as a smile when I saw him at my music lessons.

Every Thursday afternoon for two years I took clarinet lessons from Mr. Reed in his basement studio at Hauer Music. I sat in an aqua, plastic waiting-room chair, leafing through worn issues of *Life* magazine, wanting to be anywhere else but at the store. I didn't enjoy playing the clarinet, just as I didn't enjoy playing the piano, an instrument I struggled with two years earlier. But the Hauers were musicians, and it was expected that all of us kids would play an instrument or two and eventually work in the family business. I had no desire to do either.

After my lesson one Thursday, I managed to raise my eyes off the ground long enough to look up and see Bill, who took saxophone lessons from Mr. Reed right after me and maybe in that millisecond he or I said a quick "hi." And to me that was as good as saying, "I've always loved you." Thus, three years later, Bill was the only boy I could think of asking to the Turnabout Dance, an annual tradition when the girls invite the boys. It wasn't even in my sphere of thinking to go to the dance. I didn't know any boys. I didn't talk to any boys. But I felt pressured. My friends and every other girl had the courage to ask a boy. Or they already had a boyfriend. I didn't want to look even more pathetic than I already felt. So I thought at least I had some familiarity with Bill. I mean, for God's sake, I saw him every week at music lessons for how many years? It seemed like I'd known Bill forever. Yet it took me weeks, agonizing weeks, to work up the courage to make the call.

Asking a boy to a dance was a big move for me. I was unbelievably shy and felt ugly and fat and sad. I walked the halls with my head down, afraid to see what was in front of me. I scripted, wrote, and rewrote the two lines I had to recite when I made that call. When I finally did it, I blurted out, "Hi, is this Bill? This is Shary Hauer. Would you like to go to the Turnabout Dance with me?" There wasn't even a delay. No moment or two of hesitation in his response—just a resounding no.

Did I drop the phone in horror? I do not remember. I blocked it out of my mind, just like all the other painful points in my life. God knows what I expected him to say. "Oh sure, Shary, I'd love to. I've been waiting anxiously for your call. You're the only one I wanted to ask me." Heavens. Did I even *think* about preparing myself for his response?

I mumbled, "Thanks," and hung up the phone, stunned, shattered. Rejected.

Some girls would brush it off. The confident ones like Jody or Kathy would just laugh about it—"Oh well, he'll be sorry"—and move on to the next boy. And the next. Big deal. For me, it was the *biggest* deal. Another reminder that I was unattractive, unwanted, undesirable.

· ·

In 1970, when I was thirteen, our family moved fifteen miles north to a much-needed larger home in Kettering, Ohio, forcing me to abandon my last year at Incarnation and to leave friends I'd known since I was six.

In September, five of us Hauer kids enrolled at Holy Angels, in a

Catholic parish on the edge of downtown Dayton. Unlike Incarnation School, a modern, sprawling ranch-style building surrounded by acres of grass and trees in the newest suburb, Holy Angels was old and imposing. Situated next to the church, the elementary school was a beige-brick, three-story building that looked unchanged since it had been built in 1902. The tall, creaky, heavy wood front doors opened to a set of polished, beige linoleum steps and institutional prison-green walls. Only a handful of too-high windows shed narrow shafts of sunlight, and every conversation, no matter how far down the hall, echoed, bouncing off the tired walls.

I was a suburban girl who had spent seven years going to school with middle-income white kids. Holy Angels had a rough-and-tumble assemblage of blacks, Cubans, and rich white kids. The twenty-five or so girls in my class already had friends, the same best friends since first grade. I felt alone right from the start. And to make it worse, my dad registered me by my birth name: Sharmon Hauer. Mrs. Thaman, the stern seventyish English teacher with tightly permed gray hair, wire-rimmed glasses, and unsmiling lips, took roll call and called me Sharmon every day for months. Each time I cringed with horror, my head dropping down to my desk in embarrassment. Each time I heard snickers and an occasional, "Don't squeeze me, Sharmon." I was too shy and humiliated, too inward, to correct her. I hated my dad, hated him for punishing me so.

I didn't fit in from day one, and the weird name didn't help. I was an outsider—that's what I told myself. Repeatedly. Extremely self-conscious, I couldn't help but compare myself to the other girls. I didn't have pretty long hair. I was the fattest girl in the class, zitty, and one of the few who wore glasses, and I swore I was the only girl who didn't have a boyfriend. No one approached me or asked me to sit with them at lunch. I was too timid to introduce myself and sit down at one of the occupied tables.

I was overwhelmed with stimuli, automatically plugging into my teachers and fellow students, studying their looks, their whispers, their words, spoken or unspoken. I convinced myself that everyone was watching and judging the fat, introverted new girl. I did not know how to manage or filter the barrage of emotions and negative feelings flooding my system. I withdrew further.

I didn't know I needed reassurance and comfort from my parents. I didn't know to ask for it. Perhaps I did, but knew it was an impossible request. And I certainly didn't know how to reason with and comfort myself. My feelings of self-doubt and insecurity seemed all-consuming, paralyzing. But I didn't recognize these feelings back then—I thought only that I was ugly and an outsider. I crawled deeper inside myself that year, unsure of my new environment, unable to make new friends. Meanwhile, my brothers were having the time of their lives playing sports and being chased by a slew of new girls.

My cloak of sadness, according to Janet Woititz, author of *The Intimacy Struggle,* stemmed from the fact that I was an adult child who never got to be a child. I fit her description: "She did not have the experience of being spontaneous, foolish, child-like—that children normally do. She did not have an opportunity to experience fun, or even to know what fun is. This . . . makes it harder to feel free and spontaneous in any relationship."

My brothers later called my adolescent years my "wreck years." I was a wreck. When I look at family photos from those years, I see a tired, unhappy girl who could be their mother. There I stood in my ladies' aquamarine Easter dress, my frizzy hair temporarily managed in some sort of old-lady bob. I *did* look like the mother.

· ·

Despite my isolating behavior and self-consciousness, I somehow managed to capture a boy's heart. Dave was fair skinned, maybe even pale, with dark-blond hair, and kind of cute to my eighth-grade eyes. Reserved and very serious looking, he never smiled, but I suppose he'd say the same about me. He looked older than thirteen, wearing the mandatory school uniform of a white short-sleeved shirt and navy slacks. And he was smart. One day after class, he tapped my elbow on the way out the door and passed me a triangle of tightly folded 8.5-by-11 notepaper, origami style. I didn't acknowledge it, didn't know what to do with it. Dave and I never talked. What could he possibly want with me? On the school bus ride home, I carefully unwrapped the tiny parcel to read a poem about wanting to embrace my pretty eyes, printed in pen, in large, elegant letters. He must have made a mistake. Did he mean to give it to Michelle, the cute and quiet blond that sat three rows over from him? I quickly folded the paper and stuffed it into my coat pocket. It wasn't for me, that I was certain. Why would Dave send me a love note? And it was weird. He was weird I thought. When my mom and dad went away on a rare vacation together for a week, Mrs. Weller, an elderly live-in babysitter who stayed with us occasionally, came to watch us six kids. The house was unusually quiet as I sat with her in the breakfast nook at the kitchen table one afternoon. My brothers and sisters had fled an hour earlier to play basketball and race bikes in the driveway. Mrs. Weller and I lazily gazed out the windows at the vast hillside of mature oak and maple trees, the blanket of green leaves soothing and cool on that sweltering day.

"You have the prettiest complexion," she said.

I cast my eyes downward and thought, *What? What did she say?* That couldn't be right. No one had ever said anything like that to me before. I shifted uncomfortably in the chair and shook my head.

"No I don't. I have horrible skin. It's awful."

I had been going to a dermatologist every two weeks for acne treatments. I'd tried a sunlamp, the full spectrum of drugs available, plus every topical sulfuric application, none of which worked. So not only was I fat, with a hive of frizzy hair and eyeglasses, my face was landscaped with red, bumpy welts. Perhaps I had a temporary clearing on my face. *Is she crazy? Of course she is. She's old and can't see. She's imagining things.*

Little did I know that my deflecting and dismissing compliments and praise—a habit surely fueled by the Catholic canons of modesty and humility—would be the setup for a no-win love life decades later. I was blind, literally unable to see what other people saw in me. I could not own my beauty or competence or anything good about myself for that matter. Instead, all I could absorb were the negatives, my imperfection. I was a girl desperate to not feel the pain of parental neglect, and all I knew was how to reject myself and others' love.

7

The Salsa Dancer

When I was forty-four, I moved to Clearwater Beach, Florida, to fulfill my lifelong dream of living by the sea. A series of circumstances had propelled me to leave my seventeen-year corporate career in 1995 to launch my own firm in the infant executive coaching industry. A combination corporate life strategist, therapist, and cheerleader, I was now focused on helping individual leaders develop their highest potential. Finally, I had discovered a career path that felt like home. And because I was no longer tied to a desk and had the freedom to connect with my clients virtually, a seaside cottage was the perfect spot to set up shop.

While I was excited about all of the new possibilities in my life and career, I felt discombobulated, like a scared child, alone and depressed in a new place where I knew no one. I didn't have anyone to sort through my fears with, to put me at ease. Although we'd been broken up for three years, Doug and I talked on the phone every two weeks or so, and it felt good to be comforted by his calm and reassuring voice. I knew it wasn't normal to still be experiencing such painful withdrawal symptoms. After a year in Florida, the place where I intended to start my new life, I finally mustered up the courage to move on and ended all contact with him.

I networked like crazy at a half dozen business groups, found a new gym, learned to sail, explored sushi haunts with members of the Tampa Bay Sushi Society, volunteered at the food bank, and went on a couple of blind dates. I'd always been mesmerized by the fast, sexy,

Insatiable

and happy tempo of Latin dance and soon found a beginner's salsa class at a small dance studio tucked next to a roller-skating rink in an aging strip mall thirty minutes from my home.

It was a Monday night in early October, our third lesson, when our instructor, Oksana, summoned us to the dance floor. We knew the drill: men lined up in one row; women faced them. Eight women and three men, so I'd end up dancing with women—again. The tinny music from the 1980s-era boom box came on and we stumbled like toddlers, vaguely recalling the last week's lesson. Moments later, the main door creaked open, a shaft of evening light was cast in the dark ballroom, and a tall man in black sauntered in.

"One, two, three, and four," Oksana continued, eyeballing each of us.

"Yeah, a new man!" I said to the group, my eyes fixed on the new student. I was aflutter seeing a new male face. After changing into black dress shoes, he joined the men's line.

"Hi, I'm Shary. Your name?"

He seemed shy, his eyes downcast, very serious.

"Byron," he said.

"We women were just talking about how desperate we were for more men. And then, magically, you appeared."

He looked away, a faint smile across his face.

A part of me made the decision right then and there that he and I were going to be dance partners and hopefully something more. It had been four years and thirty-four days since my lips had caressed a man's—my longest dry spell—so my heart was screaming for attention and was determined to find it.

After the dance lesson was over, a few couples stayed to practice. Byron and I wobbled for an hour and then walked outside to our cars. He was six foot one, with thin, light-brown hair, hazel eyes, and a pleasant face, and as I engaged him in a conversation all about him, I became more excited about the possibility of us. He was intelligent, fluent in German, and a chemical engineer with patents. He had invented an apparatus for cooling a light beam. I had no idea that light beams needed cooling. And he had designed a device to generate reactive ions. He lived in Texas, was in Florida as a consultant on a special light-beam assignment, a lover of antiquarian books, and as

96

passionate about learning Latin dance as I was. Oh my God. I was smitten already.

"How long will you be in town?" I asked.

"Just until tomorrow," he said.

"It'd sure be great to practice some more. When will you be back?"

"In two weeks. Do you want to get together then?"

We set a date for dinner and dancing on the Saturday night he was to return and said good-bye. I drove home, singing and shaking to the *Salsa Caliente* CD I had turned up to full volume, juiced, making a list of all I had to do to get ready for our date: buy a new seductive dress, dancing shoes, definitely new lacy lingerie, perfume, bubble bath, and maybe a sexy nightgown or two. The list went on.

· ·

We met for dinner at a tiny sushi restaurant in Safety Harbor, a quaint village on Tampa Bay. He seemed uncomfortable. I had forgotten how reserved and serious he was; I had built him up in my mind so much as a great conversationalist. True to form, I became the interviewer to encourage him to open up, asking him about his life in Texas, his work. He responded politely but didn't seem to have the ability or desire to reciprocate.

Halfway through our dinner, I sat back, sipping my hot ginger tea, feeling exhausted. His shyness was overwhelming. But I didn't know it as shyness then. Rather I interpreted it as nonchalance about being with me. But we managed through. I would always burn miles of energy rescuing a bad evening in the name of being with a man. It never occurred to me to say, "Listen, you know this isn't going to work out" or even "I've got a headache. I'm sorry, I can't go dancing." To cut it off then. I didn't have the capacity to recognize that I was doing all the work. To recognize that I was miserable. To recognize that this guy wasn't relationship material and move on.

Instead, I was an expert at plowing ahead. I'd always managed to muscle through awkward conversations, hungry and determined to be with a man no matter how excruciating. It's not so bad, I told myself. There have been worse. And even though I learned that Byron was battling his ex-wife for custody of his ten-year-old daughter, financially destitute, fighting over a contract with a former business partner, and recently laid off, I chose to overlook the whole mess. I was ravenous for male attention, and I was going to get it, even if it was from this limping, wounded soul who happened to live nine hundred miles away. Lower my standards? Yes. Settle for less? Always. Find a fixer-upper? My specialty. As long as I still did not get—really *get*—how badly I treated myself or how my vast hunger was the source of all of the angst, misery, and heartbreak I'd experienced in my love life, it was easier for me to remain ignorant of my underlying issues. I wasn't able to make those connections yet.

We arrived at the Penguin Dance Club, an old-school all-Latin club, at about 9:30, early for the Latin crowd. We stood on the sidelines, drinking from our plastic cups of chardonnay, watching dancers starting to stream in. I was buoyant: the music, the lights, with a new man who liked to dance. But Byron looked nervous, studying the dancers as if they were a chemistry experiment, his brow furrowed. I stood close to him, swaying my hips, eager to get out on the dance floor. An hour later, he finally asked me to dance and took my hand, the floor now mobbed with couples wrapped around one another, mamboing. The only gringos, we found an out-of-the-way corner to brush up on our salsa moves. We assumed the basic step position, and Byron started counting the beats out loud, very slowly, one, two, three, and four. One, two, three, and four. His eyes locked to his feet, counting. No fun, no laughter, only serious concentration. I was the cheerleader. "You're doing great," I said. "Look how much you already learned in our lessons." I willed him courage and a zip in his salsa moves.

After dancing, on our way out the door, we saw a flyer promoting private dance lessons with Latin dancing pros Simone and José. Group lessons on Monday; private lessons on Thursdays. Why not? As he was returning to Texas in a few days, I offered to make the arrangements and schedule lessons for when he came back to Florida.

Communication between his visits was sparse. He didn't do e-mail and hated talking on the phone. It drove me crazy. After one date and more to come, I expected some warmth and connection, a hint of romantic interest. I detected none.

Two weeks later we had our first individual lessons and then met for coffee and dessert afterward at a café down the street. He was still tentative, answering my questions cordially but not offering much more. By our third dance date, I had given up. I made up my mind that he would be a dance partner only, and only occasionally. I decided to stop hoping for a romantic relationship. He wasn't fun to be with. By the time our private lesson rolled around, I regretted having made the arrangements. I was tired of making an effort with this man.

But just when I had made my resolution, he surprised me by calling the evening before our next class and saying, "I want to make you dinner. How about Chinese? It's my specialty." At 5:00 p.m. on a Saturday in early December, he knocked on my front door, loaded down with an elaborate outdoor wok setup and a shopping list. He unpacked his gear, and we drove off to the produce market to stock up on bundles of vegetables for stir-fry. Back home, he helped me strategize on how to get my new cat, an abandoned female calico named Tiggie, to settle down. She cried incessantly when I put her outside. I didn't know how to handle a needy cat. He was the cat whisperer, calming her with his soft strokes and tender words. I poured us a glass of wine and we started on dinner, chopping the vegetables side by side. I loved the picture of a couple in love cooking together. It's what I'd always wanted. And seeing him assume command, taking charge with the dinner, the shopping, and Tiggie, made me take notice. I wanted a strong, in-control man. Plus, he was far more relaxed and lighthearted than he'd ever been. It was turning into an enjoyable evening. Still, I had recalibrated—we were to be friends, just dancing buddies.

After dinner and dancing, he ran to the supermarket to get supplies to make me his signature chocolate-covered strawberries. At midnight he suggested we go outside to the backyard to stargaze. I grabbed a couple of blankets from the linen closet, and we lay in the grass looking up at the sky, the palm-tree fronds gently swaying in the light breeze. Our shoulders touched as he quietly pointed to constellations I'd never heard of. Drowsy from the wine, I closed my eyes, and was nearly lulled to sleep by the chirping crickets. Suddenly, I felt his lips on mine. I shot right up.

"Where did that come from?" I asked, stunned.

"I've been wanting to do it for months," he said. "But I was afraid you would turn me down."

Oh my. Such fear. A grown man afraid of being rejected. But his lips were soft. Perfect. Here was the man I'd been hungry for after all. We latched onto each other, necking for an hour or so before going inside and creating a makeshift bed on my oversized red couch. We snuggled and caressed and kissed until 4:00 a.m., when he lumbered out the door.

I couldn't sleep, keyed up with adrenaline. What an evening! Shopping and making dinner together, dancing, delicious wine, sweet chocolate-covered strawberries, lying side by side under the stars, kissing for hours. It was a page from a script, one of my imagined romance vignettes. The setting, the tastes, the aromas and colors, the music—all the things I loved. Romance. My cocaine. I knew I'd be up for days.

I was resurrected! How energized and happy I was—I officially had a new man in my life! It's normal to feel exhilarated with a new potential lover. What's not normal is the extent to which I did not feel fully alive unless I was with a romantic partner. When I entered a new relationship, what I *believed* to be a relationship, the sun came out again. I felt powerful, confident, purposeful. I laughed more. I could think more quickly. But in between relationships, during the dry spells, I felt lost, anchorless.

Byron had to return to Texas in two days and wouldn't be back to Florida until early January, after the holiday season. An entire month before I would see him again. What was I going to do? Now that I thought of us as a couple, I needed constant connection and reinforcement: *Do you care about me? Have you been thinking of me? Do you want me?* I needed him close, expected him to call or write every few days. But once he got back to his life and problems in Texas, he was nearly mute. I tried to refocus my energy on my clients and business, but instead I channeled it all toward the next time with him. I needed to lose ten pounds before he returned. I stocked the kitchen with his favorites: cabernet sauvignon, and tins of homemade ginger snaps and black licorice. I decorated the guest room with a new bedspread and pillows. I wanted to make myself feel and look fabulous: I had my hair cut and colored, my nails manicured and pedicured, and my body waxed. I spent days away from work, primping the house and myself, preparing for his arrival.

· ❧ ·

By the time he walked through my door at midnight in mid-January, wearing a jean jacket, hiking boots, and a huge tired smile, I pounced on him like a jaguar in heat. Our clothes were off in seconds. It had been more than four years since I had made love. I was on fire with his warm, taut, naked body covering mine, his cushiony lips tickling my ear. "I have been waiting to be with you for months," he whispered. What a rush seeing the longing in his eyes. My skin vibrated under his tender touch, softening as his arms encircled and secured me. I was euphoric. My movie-script version of the perfect new relationship had unfolded. The sex wasn't especially memorable. It never was for me. That wasn't the focus. I needed and got a hit off his passion, his desire for me, him wanting me. For the first time in years, I felt like the vibrant, whole woman I was meant to be. Finally, at forty-four, I had something that felt permanent.

As Byron was at a critical juncture with his Florida consulting project, he'd be staying in town longer—we'd have three glorious weeks together, and I was ecstatic. I put my mothering instinct into overdrive, masterminding a series of romantic scenarios and creating a cozy nest at my beach cottage. Knowing his life was in disarray, I wanted nothing more than to please and distract him from his troubles. Ocean-scented candles glowing, freshly cut hibiscus arrangements placed just so, we comforted each other and made love tenderly in my fluffy-pillowed bed. From time to time, we reluctantly left the cottage to walk on the winter beach, then returned to warm our chilly bodies with each other and mugs of hot cocoa.

After work one evening, I waited for him in the laboratory parking lot, my car loaded with fixings for a sunset beach picnic: salads and appetizers from Guppy's—my favorite seafood place, blankets, wine, homemade cookies, and lots of votive candles. He ran out of the building to my car, jumped in with several shopping bags, and hugged me. "I've missed you," he said, holding my face next to his. Like an eager kid on Christmas morning, he presented a bundle of gifts: a gorgeous Thai cookbook, massage oil, a book of *Far Side* cartoons, and citrus body lotion. We stayed after sunset, lying on the sand wrapped tightly in blankets, sipping wine, kissing, and caressing. A comet streaked across the cloudless sky, and we both burst out, "Oh my God, did you see that?" We sat up amazed, hoping for a curtain call. I had never seen a comet. I took it as a sign, an affirmation from the heavens: this, us, was magical.

On one of our long, morning beach walks, we gathered sea treasures piled on the sugary white sand—starfish, urchins, and horseshoe-crab skeletons. As I walked off to a dune to search for sand dollars, he came up beside me and pulled out a foot-long egg casing—from a whelk— from behind his back and lunged it in front of me like a jack-in-the-box, laughing. I jumped back and fell into the sand, giggling. *How wonderful this is, he is,* I thought. Finally, a man who appreciated the quiet and natural beauty of this place as much as I did. I was so happy walking hand in hand, exploring my favorite place on earth with a man I loved. It was an idyllic honeymoon with a deep, soulful man I had first written off as boring and uncommunicative.

But one morning in bed, toward the end of his stay I found myself in a tense discussion with him about having children. He wanted to raise another one. I was forty-four, past my baby-making prime, and I had no interest in having a child at that stage. Right then I had a moment of clarity and realized how many differences we had. He was unable to access and share deeper thoughts and feelings. I lived in the realm of feelings. He saw his world through a dingy lens: bad stuff happens, life is unfair, people are vindictive. He was fearful, reticent, unsure of himself, and attracted to strong-willed people like his ex-wife, his ex-boss, and now me, who overpowered and overwhelmed him. He was struggling with money and finding work; I was successful with a good income. He seemed to attract problems—so much in his life was unsettled, unraveling. I saw the world and people in sunnier, more hopeful ways: look at the blessings, the gifts we have. That should have been the end of the story.

Looking back at my journal many years later, I saw that I had written about our incompatibilities and the wrongness of our relationship from the beginning. Again, the truth always landed on the page. But I was unable to absorb or process it. The needier Jekyll part of me ruled. Despite every reason in the book that Byron and I were not a good, healthy match, I claimed I was "in love." I argued like a top lawyer in my head about why Byron was right for me. Despite the mountain of incompatibilities and red flags, I still justified the relationship. I embellished, distorted the rightness of us, because I wanted, needed a relationship. Because I was ready for a partner and marriage. Because I believed that everyone is fixable.

I preferred to see what Bryon could be, that he was gleaming with possibility. He was brilliant, professionally respected, gentle, and kind. All he needed was some time to sort through his issues. He'd had a setback, that's all. He'd find a great job soon. And the situation with his ex-wife and daughter—that would resolve itself. I was sure. And I was committed to doing anything to make us better. I vowed to be more patient with Byron's troubled life. I prayed to be less needy and more loving. My blindness was stupefying. I had absolutely no ability to filter and see the truth: this relationship was DOA, not bliss. How I could get so distorted in love was such a befuddlement to me. But now I can see it more clearly. I simply wanted to feel loved. And I vehemently feared being a woman on her own. I had fallen into the same trap as all the other women who have bought into the Cinderella and Snow White notion that we are incomplete without a man in our life, conditioned to believe that our lives lack joy, value, and purpose if we are alone. According to Dr. Penelope Russianoff, author of *Why Do I Think I Am Nothing Without a Man?*, women who are "desperately dependent" are women who feel adrift and "make men, or the lack of a man, the major focus in her life." Who was I, I asked myself, without a man by my side?

I was terrified that Byron would run away and abandon me after I had invested what I thought was my complete love and trust in him. I couldn't fathom tearing my insides out again with the horror of another breakup. I was desperate to get it right this time. I'd deny, overlook, and minimize just about any fault just to temporarily experience that glorious feeling of being wanted. I couldn't yet see that I had a serious problem, an addiction. I didn't see that my insatiable hunger for male attention attracted men who were as wounded as I was.

The one thing I wasn't completely blind to was the emerging sense that I didn't love myself enough. In some remote place in my heart, I was grasping that my dependence on Byron, any man, to feed me love was wrong. Even though I had made a commitment to cherish myself more after breaking up with Doug, the fact that I got in so deep, so fast, with Byron, a man with a boatload of issues, was a sure sign that I was far more alienated from loving myself than I imagined.

· ·

Byron said he couldn't wait to see me again in three weeks, when he planned to return and wrap up his project in Clearwater.

"Call me, please? Just to let me know you arrived home safely," I said.

He picked up his worn duffel bag and swung the shoulder strap across his chest. "I'll try," he said. "You know I've got so much ugliness I have to sort through. I can't commit to much of anything right now."

We clutched one another and said our weepy airport good-byes. He returned to Texas—and then went incommunicado, as if he had vanished. I didn't hear from him for three days. I was a wreck. I tortured myself, obsessing about what went wrong. But by day four, I was angry. *I deserve better treatment than this. Who does he think he is? How could anyone do this to me?* The logical thing to do would be to call to see if he was alright. But I didn't want to bother him— he told me he was going to be buried with work and home projects. Still, I couldn't stop thinking about him. Every time the phone rang, I jumped up, hoping to see his name on caller ID. Too stunned, too hurt to call, I was immobilized. I wept and rewound each of our recent conversations, struggling for an explanation, a shard of hope.

Another week went by. Meanwhile, I tried to shove the shell shock out of my voice and to replace it with perkiness when I was on the phone with my coaching clients. In between calls, I comforted myself by reading don Miguel Ruiz's *The Mastery of Love* repeatedly and by absorbing soothing words from my dear friends Kathy and Sheila. The best balm was taking a long-weekend trip to lusty New Orleans with my sister, and as I always did after a heartbreak, I committed to more volunteer hours with Tampa Bay Harvest, Neighborly Seniors, and the Homeless Emergency Project, helping those who were truly suffering. When I finally tamed my tears and called to check on him, the call went straight to voice mail. Three times. I didn't leave a message. Then I panicked, fearing that he had committed suicide, was ill, or had been in an accident.

It's normal to grieve the loss of a relationship, but most people move through the emotions of hurt, pain, sorrow, and heartache and come to feel better in a reasonable time frame. But as with many love addicts, I got stuck and went through an anguishing withdrawal. My descent from Fantasy Island to icy reality was a jarring body slam. For weeks I was enveloped in a tsunami of anxiety, panic, insomnia, obsession, rage, and despair. "There's no difference . . . between an addict coming off heroin and a woman coming off an obsessive relationship," says love addiction expert Robin Norwood. How right she is. Searing rejection and abandonment scalded my spirit. Just as I felt resurrected with a new man, when he left, I died. I felt purposeless. I didn't feel charming or beautiful or joyful anymore. Just dead. I was drowning in deep hopelessness: *Will I ever get it right?* Although I didn't yet recognize that I was in a self-destructive pattern of repeating bad relationships, I did think of myself as a failure in love. I had been with John, Patrick, Doug, and now Byron. Eighteen years of my life had passed, and all I had to show for it was a pile of collapsed relationships.

But what I knew deep inside and unconsciously blocked out was that Byron had told me he needed some space. He had implored me, truthfully. He had said he needed to get through his stacked-up life, had too many crises to deal with. But I didn't like that version of the story, the true version. My life storyline was abandonment, and apparently I needed to keep stoking it: men abandon me. They flee. I'm unlovable.

In retrospect, it seemed I was more addicted to the pain and suffering than I was to love. My only reference to love came from romance stories and movies, especially those of unrequited love. The dramatic, tragic tales of love. I bawled for days after watching the priest Ralph de Bricassart spend his entire life tormented, pining for his forbidden lover, Meggie Cleary, in *The Thorn Birds*. And I could literally feel Ryan O'Neal's wrenching pain as he said good-bye to his terminally ill young wife, played by Ali MacGraw, in *Love Story*.

I didn't know back then that it was my responsibility to manage my suffering. I hadn't the tools or insight yet to cease the incessant pain and anguish of abandonment. I didn't yet see how I was contributing, perpetuating, fanning the flames by feeding and indulging in my anguish. Suffering, pain, hurt, and anger were familiar—they were what I knew, what I projected. I didn't realize that I manifested them over and over again.

It had been almost six weeks since Byron had returned to Texas, and I still hadn't heard a peep from him. After scripting for days what I wanted to say, I summoned the courage to call him again. This time, I left an upbeat but serious message saying that I was thinking about him and hoped he was alright. Hours later, while I was in a deep sleep, he resurfaced. I received five after-midnight voice-mail messages explaining how he felt his world of woes had been bringing our relationship down. He couldn't handle it. So he had disappeared. Had gone to Mexico. "I'm sorry for being inconsiderate. I've been thinking about you. I miss you," he said. By that point, all I could feel was pity. The romance high was punctured. I sent prayers his way and moved on.

Yet a month later, I flip-flopped. Remembering Byron's birthday was coming up in April, I hatched a plan: wouldn't it be wonderful to invite him to the beach for a weekend celebration—a gift of much-needed peace and happiness? He loved the warm Gulf of Mexico waters, the serenity of my desolate tip of Clearwater Beach. Certainly he needed a break from his troubles. A few days in the sun and surf might give him a fresh perspective.

I'd send a playful invitation to a private birthday party at the beach, fly him in from Texas on a Friday morning, and grant him a treasure chest of wishes, including magical sunsets, sunrises, walking, wading, swimming with the dolphins, his favorite cake, and me, dancing a special birthday striptease. As charitable as I thought I was, I craved only one thing—another hit, another high, mainlining his love and affection. The allure of another lustful beach weekend was intense. The longing to re-create the dreamy illusion of love was all that mattered. Thank God my longtime business and life coach Meryl intervened to show me the futility of my plan before I humiliated myself. In matters of the heart, Meryl had always been a wise beacon for me, and I had reached out to her more than once in the prior few weeks to calm my hysteria.

"You got the best of him, Shary," she said. "He is laden with problems. Why would you settle for someone who is staggering through life when you are soaring?"

It's exactly what I needed to hear. Like a child sticking a dirty pebble in my mouth, I needed to hear, "Put that down! Don't eat that rock. Ick!" Once again, I could see the lengths I went to justify any relationship, no matter how wrong it was. I could itemize all the reasons the relationship was bad for me and still pursue it. Why in the world would I settle for someone so far off my radar of desired qualities? And worse, this time I was willing to pay for it. Yes, I would have been a gigolo—flying Byron in for the weekend to satisfy my voracious addiction.

Once Meryl helped me see that Byron's birthday trip wasn't a healthy proposition, I never spoke to him again. But, out of the blue, a month later, I received an e-mail from him—his first and only one to me. In it he apologized for hurting me, for causing me so much agony. "I'm sure this breakup is as painful for you as it is for me," he wrote.

It was too little, too late. I wasn't in pain anymore. By that time, my heart was already gearing up for my next fix.

8
Feeding Frenzy

During the spring and summer months following Byron's retreat and the end of our six-month relationship, I poured energy into my flourishing executive coaching business, invested in spiritual growth, volunteered, planned a summer hiking vacation in the Greek Islands, and made new friends at belly-dancing class, sushi-making class, and windsurfing lessons. My love life was not as productive. I was forty-five and still single, with not a prospect in sight. I wasn't desperate or panicky, only discouraged, hoping being partnerless was just a temporary blip. In some way, I think forty-five marked an unconscious halfway point in my love life: a pause to say, get on with it!! A few well-intentioned friends attempted to set me up on blind dates that ended up going nowhere. Except for a daily 5:00 a.m. gym workout, weekend outings with girlfriends, and evening walks on the beach, I lived a pretty cloistered life. I worked alone in my home office from sunup to sundown and traveled for business every other week or two. And in a resort beach town, not a business or urban center, the pickings were slim. The occasional man I did meet was fifteen or twenty years older, freshly divorced and relocated to Florida, with an itch to christen his new single life with a younger babe. I figured my best chance of meeting a respectable man was in an airport terminal racing to catch my next flight. Or online.

The week before Thanksgiving 2002, dateless for nine months, I reluctantly joined Match.com. I knew the rules: Don't use my primary e-mail account. Don't give out my address or phone numbers. Always have an initial date in the daytime, preferably for coffee. Be aware of misrepresentations and exaggerations. I heeded the precautions and dove in.

Jim was one of the first gents I met online. Ten years older, overly self-deprecating, he didn't appeal to me physically and was needy to boot. But we had a mutual appreciation for wit and creative writing, and our e-mail repartee was great entertainment. And I was attracted to Jim's Buddhist leanings, his love of the arts, and, more than anything else, his flattery. I was the Energizer Bunny incarnate; my upbeat zest for life was way off the charts, he said, and I had missed my calling as the female Dave Barry. Jim's praise and adoration were juicy bait luring me closer. Although I was pretty certain I had no romantic interest in him, once again, that didn't seem to matter. I knew he wanted me. My craving for male attention would be fed aplenty with Jim.

We first met on a gloomy December Sunday afternoon at Starbucks. I walked in to see a balding man wearing glasses and head-to-toe denim sitting alone in the corner.

"Jim?" I asked.

He stood. "Wow, don't I feel like a slug. You're dressed like a million bucks."

It was my normal winter wardrobe: black dress slacks, black turtleneck, and a scarf. I always had a scarf thrown around my neck. I wasn't a jeans and T-shirt kind of woman; I didn't even own a pair of jeans. I was used to hearing comments about being overdressed or people thinking I was from New York.

Although Jim was in great shape, a daily runner, and pleasant looking, our first meeting confirmed my earlier suspicions that I would not be attracted to him. But our conversations were easy and comfortable, just like talking to a girlfriend. And unlike many of the men I'd conversed with online who were two-dimensional—just work and golf—or were retired and looking to hang out with a woman full time, Jim was a multifaceted doer with a crammed social calendar who knew all the weekend goings-on in Tampa Bay. He loved tasting life tapas-style as much as I did. I'd written in my e-mails and said just moments before that I was looking to meet more like-minded pals—code for *I'm not interested in you as a lover*.

However, an hour later, shivering and standing next to my car, ready to say good-bye, Jim said, "I'd like to see you again. I'm interested in pursuing a relationship with you."

Oh Lord, I thought. *Wasn't I clear about what I wanted?* "Well, I'm really just looking for companions and buddies right now," I reiterated—not realizing then that this was my standard safeguard story, my attempt to keep men distant when closeness was all I ached for. It was the same as when I told Patrick and Doug in our first month of dating that we were in a transition relationship. I didn't know then I was lying or deceiving. I honestly didn't. I didn't yet grasp that I was a bipolar lover: simultaneously craving and repelling intimacy and commitment.

"I want a girlfriend, not another friend," he said, pausing for a couple of moments. "But you never can have too many friends." He smiled, pecked me on my cheek, and opened my car door. "How about lunch and the gallery hop in Saint Pete Saturday?"

"That sounds fun. I've never been."

Two days after our Saturday date, I invited Jim over for dinner and a beach walk. Our conversation continued to flow effortlessly. Like me, he had an opinion on a vast number of topics, namely the ineptitude of corporate management, spirituality, and Match.com activity. By date three, I unconsciously registered that he would be a lovely playmate—a regular, steady, always-willing puppy of a guy that I could manage and manipulate to my heart's content.

The first time he kissed me, I couldn't feel his lips; his mouth lay dormant under mine, anemic. I politely pulled away. But the following week at his place, after emphatically restating my intentions—"I am not interested in a romantic relationship with you"—I surprised myself by reciprocating his kisses with the will and vigor of a champion boxer in the ring for an all-night match. We went full-bore into a petting session that lasted until after midnight. His kissing hadn't improved at all. But after a few caresses and warm kisses, my addicted self yawned awake with the heady chemical rush of romance and desire. We saw each other two, three, sometimes four times a week, for beach walks, cooking sessions, wine tasting, and late-night groping and conversations, trying to top one another in our new game: you're not going to believe the crazy I heard from on Match.com this week.

· ☙ ·

While Jim and I dated, I continued to search and flirt on Match.com, captivating men with my charming and engaging e-mails. With its legions of "qualified" single men in a twenty-mile radius of my home, Match.com was my new catnip. I went into a feeding frenzy, getting and sending winks and messages to an in-box full of men. There was Les, who intrigued me with his formal messages harkening romantic medieval times. And when I read John's profile, my WOW-meter zinged. Articulate, upbeat, an entrepreneur with an airplane who was launching an adventure business in the Bahamas. Wow! I envisioned jetting off with Indiana Jones to the islands for the weekend to snorkel the pristine Caribbean and to gorge on just-caught spiny lobster. We met for a sushi lunch, and immediately I smelled his nervousness and discomfort. I joked, laughed, attempted to make him feel comfortable, as he was literally sweating through his entire meal. And he was crass, wiping his sweat, his nose, holding his chopsticks like a caveman—not necessarily the gentleman I expected. All bets were off when he had no qualms admitting that his ambition was to be a corporate husband to a hardworking sugar mama. The conversation ceased until he asked, "How do you want to handle the bill . . . split?" *How rude,* I thought. *If you have to ask, I'll give you another option: I'll pay for it. Get a little practice having your sugar mama take care of you.* That's how I handled it. Another bubble burst.

Another chap, whose Match.com handle was His Majesty James Bond, sent gallant poetry. And there was Bill, a pleasant retail buyer with too-black dyed hair. There was the Dutch PhD, the Frenchman who stated his undying love, and a half dozen others, none of whom got beyond the first phone conversation or coffee date.

Throughout my pursuit, there was Jim. Good ol' Jim. My buddy. A buddy I flirted with, kissed, and made out with, endlessly contradicting myself and confusing him. "Every night it's a roller-coaster ride," he said. No, yes. Yes, no. We're friends only—only to be lying half-dressed on his couch the next night. I blamed my loose and manipulative behavior on hormones; *I'm in heat,* I told myself. I didn't make the addiction connection back then. It wasn't hormones at all. It was my greedy hunger for attention, affection, adoration that drove me to flit, play, flirt, and cajole these men. I wanted a buddy and a pal? Hardly. That was another form of denial, my way of keeping my heart from getting involved and hurt again. I constantly justified the fling with Jim, telling myself I was a very affectionate woman who loved touching and being touched. What was wrong with that? Looking back, I am amazed at how I defended my behavior, saying all relationships were about learning, about growing—spiritual tests. True. But not the whole truth: I needed a fix, and any old thing would do. I was a selfish, manipulative addict who would do anything—well, almost anything; I didn't sleep with Jim—to secure romantic attention and adoration.

What I was able to articulate in my journal at the time but not yet face was at the core of my game playing and addiction. It was my great wall of fear. I feared success. I feared being disliked. I feared being dumped. I feared missing out on the life I had dreamed about—life with a wonderful partner who shared my love of travel and serving others. I had an ever-creeping fear of being alone. I already felt alone. My family—my parents and five siblings—had their obligations, spouses, and children. I was simply scared to death of being alone. Thus I clung to fantasies and the possibility of being rescued, no matter how wrong a guy was for me.

While I trolled on Match.com, my innocent fantasies comforted me. If a handsome man smiled at me, like the overly flirtatious guy at the gym I'd seen almost every day for the past year, I leaped to imagining that he wanted to be with only me—until I found out he had a wife. I fantasized and created possibilities in my head constantly although I had no idea that was what I was doing. Concocting scenarios of ideal love was so ingrained in me that I wasn't able to see the reality others saw. When it came to men, rose-colored glasses were pinned to my head permanently—until another bubble burst, when I found the young, hot sailing instructor I had lusted over had a girlfriend or that my ex-husband, John, had been sleeping with the intern. I had no choice but to face the immense amount of time I wasted thinking about and hoping, looking, wishing for a partner to make me feel significant again.

What I only recently have come to understand is that daydreaming made me feel better. It wasn't just being with a man who adored me that I was addicted to. I got a fix from innocent fantasizing. The chemical change in my body, that stirring of new possibility and joy, the dream of magical love—that's what I was addicted to.

It would have been too easy to keep seeing Jim—he was at my beck and call, an always ready and plentiful source to refuel my attention and affection deficit. But I felt increasingly guilty for manipulating a nice, innocent guy. I needed to detox, remove myself from the temptation to paw and use a man. So, four months after we met, we agreed to a "friends-only" arrangement. For the first time in my life, I was able to adhere to the terms. That was a pretty big deal for me, and I even surprised myself. Perhaps I had made more progress than I was giving myself credit for.

At the beginning of the New Year, 2003, three months after joining Match.com, I met Vernie online. He said he couldn't contain his excitement when he read my first message—yes, I sent as many as I received. "I had to read your narrative twice," he wrote. "I could not believe it the first time through, how much of a match we are! Please, you are not to write to another!!!!!!:) :) :)" I loved certain and decisive men, men with swagger and confidence whose words rippled with testosterone, like John and Patrick. In our subsequent e-mails and phone conversations, Vernie and I laughed nonstop about ridiculous things. I howled when he told me how he had to make a sales call in full business attire at Paradise Lakes, the local nudist resort. He had demonstrated the merits of industrial turf pesticides to a trio of naked people, his eyes never diverting from the grass below. Within our first two phone calls, I had already formulated an image of the Vernie I wanted him to be: a man dedicated to his fascinating career—he was a horticulturist—devoted to his extended family, particularly his three young nephews and nieces, and steadfast in his Catholicism. I liked that he was a secure, successful, quiet ex-Navy man who didn't need to prove a thing to anyone. I envisioned enchanting nights meandering the Gulf on the stately thirty-foot cruiser he had lovingly restored, followed by a fireside nightcap in his gorgeous waterfront home.

We first met for a drink at a popular bayside restaurant in Indian Rocks Beach on a late Friday afternoon in breezy January. He was a gentleman, and conversation flowed. But I wasn't physically attracted to him—I preferred tall men, and Vernie was just five foot nine. We exchanged commonalities and the requisite data points: I was the oldest of six kids; he was the middle of six kids. "You're the saint, and I'm the warped one," he said. We both chuckled, and we made a date to meet for dinner the next week in downtown Saint Petersburg.

I invited him to my place for dinner the following Tuesday night, when he jokingly told me he was an accomplished Italian chef and that he was bringing his favorite cookbook, *The Art of Cooking Naked*. I laughed and told him I didn't cook Italian and certainly not naked but that I hoped grouper on the grill and a great bottle of red wine would suffice. During a lovely dinner on the porch, I learned that Vernie was a poet, had had a book published, was a master woodworker, and was an expressive, wise, humble, and loving guy. This was the part of courtship I loved most—getting to know someone, sensing his attraction, imagining the next date and the possibility of us. Our evening ended with a gentlemanly good-night kiss on the lips.

By week four, Vernie wanted to know my business travel schedule for the next several months, to plan our dates and potential trips together, he said. I didn't even know this guy, and he wanted to manage my schedule already? When I sensed a man moving too quickly, making assumptions, I froze. The same thing had happened with John, Patrick, and Doug. I desperately hoped for their attention, yet when they came on strong in the first few weeks, I couldn't handle it. I feared being engulfed; I know that now. I had a form of emotional claustrophobia. I feared feeling overwhelmed by Doug's and John's and Patrick's emotional expectations of me—residue from being neglected by and isolated from those I had put my trust in, my mom and dad.

With Vernie, I conveniently "forgot" to bring my day planner to our next date. When we shared more details about our relationship pasts, he said he had dated and been engaged to a bisexual. As if it was everyday dinner conversation, his voice turned soft and wistful when he described the threesomes they had had. I didn't know how to respond. I was nowhere near as sexually adventurous. The idea of a threesome was a huge turnoff, not appealing to me in the least.

As we became more comfortable with one another, our conversations seemed to turn sarcastic, with an occasional jab from left field. When I made an innocent crack about men behaving badly in their fifties, an "I'm going to smack you" flew out of his mouth. He smiled and I laughed uncomfortably. "I'm joking," he said. *What a weird thing to joke about,* I thought. But my thought was just that—a quick glance and not another second of consideration. Like a wisp of a breeze that momentarily brushed my arm but did not linger. It was the same way I had responded when he told me he was the warped one and had been engaged to a bisexual. The information went in, but it was ignored. Desperate to be loved, desperate for a relationship, I went to extreme lengths to ignore what was right in front of me.

One Saturday night he invited me to his place for a home-cooked dinner he had been planning for weeks. Chilled glasses of pinot grigio in our hands, we walked through the lofty space with soaring walls and expansive windows overlooking the glistening bay. Vernie caressed the beautiful mahogany bookshelves he had handcrafted and pointed out the grain detail of the staircase he had just refinished.

"It's a magnificent space, so open, so comfortable," I said, scanning the room.

"What's that handprint on the ceiling?" I asked, puzzled, looking up.

"I'm going to put a handprint on you," he said, laughing. I mumbled something like, "Oh really?" and quickly changed the subject.

After dinner, I helped him clean the dishes, he poured another glass of wine, and we started to make our way to the living room. Standing side by side, he reached for my waist and drew me close to him. I leaned in anticipating our first tender kiss. Suddenly, he forced his mouth hard, urgently against mine, pressing my lips and my teeth, his hands pawing my breasts.

"What are you doing? What was that?" I jumped back, shaking.

"What, what are you talking about?" he asked.

"That kiss was way too aggressive," I said. "Inappropriate."

"Did you want me to be more aggressive?" he asked.

What?! More aggressive? What's wrong with him? Is he delusional? Drunk? I've got to leave. Now. And I did.

At 1:00 a.m., with more than my quota of wine, I drove the hour-long ride home, cautiously climbing the mountainous four-mile Sunshine Skyway Bridge, both hands gripping the steering wheel, all the way thanking God I had left his house when I did.

The following Monday morning, he called my office.

"You'll be glad to know that because of you, I went back to therapy," he said.

"Oh, really," I said, sitting up in my chair. "For what?"

"My therapist wants to know if you have had a history of abuse. Your comment about the kiss being too aggressive suggested to him that you have been abused."

I laughed. *What? You've got to be kidding me. He's twisting this around, saying I have a problem, and now he's in cahoots with his "therapist"?*

"Vernie, your therapist said that? Really? I have not been abused. Your kiss was too aggressive. I'm glad you're back in therapy. That's a good thing."

A week went by with no contact. I was relieved, thankful. A few days later, he called.

"I know I've been distant. I've been meaning to tell you," he said, "for me, there's a difference between sex and lovemaking. I like rough sex."

I remained quiet. I didn't know how to respond. Oh, that explains it, my mind rapidly rewinding his violent references over the previous few months.

He continued to describe scenarios involving walls, restraints, and spanking, telling me what he liked and expected from his partner. For once, I was silent, resisting the urge to yell, "You sicko," and slam the phone down. An hour later he forwarded me an e-mail with the message, "What do you think of this?" I opened the attachment: a photo of a woman with flaming-red hair standing spread eagle in full black leather dominatrix togs, whip included. I swallowed and quickly deleted his message. Even though I wanted no more contact, I was flooded with a surge of disappointment. The end of another possibility. Another check in my loss column. I fell into a slump.

• •

Only years later did I understand that I had toyed with these guys. I knew right from the start that I was not interested in getting serious with them. It had nothing to do with me wanting them. It was *all* about them wanting me. I sought only the arousal of being pursued and courted. I defended myself in my head: *It's fun. What's wrong with a little companionship? I'm meeting new friends.* Again, I obliterated the boundaries between friends and lovers. Although I made love to neither Jim nor Vernie, I certainly didn't hold to my friends-only mantra. I baited and then retreated like a con artist, all to receive affection and warmth, to feel special, to be held and caressed and lavished. It was a game I played unwittingly to tantalize and feed my narcissistic hunger. Back then, I didn't feel guilty in the least bit.

I thought of my few months with Jim, Vernie, and the other assorted Match.com dates as my personal Mardi Gras, a reward for months of brutal work and travel. I needed a break from my routine and I took one. I got intoxicated being with a different man every night of the week. I'd never had three dates in a week—a record. For the first time in my life, I felt confident, emboldened with men. It was fun, tiring, exhilarating. Fueled by adrenaline and the allure of more and more attention and romance, I didn't have time to assess, process. The racing-energy, flirty, laughing, loving-life, no-sleep, losing-weight, anxious state I was in was akin to the frenetic high of cocaine.

At the time, I was clueless that the constant stream of cyber attention ensnared me. For some love addicts, online dating sites are like a Willy Wonka–sized store where all the candy they could possibly want is free. With hundreds, thousands of candidates from which to choose, love addicts can shop for partners for hours, sometimes days on end, becoming addicted to online dating. With one click, an addict can wink and chat and e-mail and fantasize and have the illusion of a thriving dating life when in reality there is nothing of substance. My obsessiveness definitely escalated online. When I did not receive a reply to one of my winks or hear back from a guy who seemed so hot and heavy the day before, or when I noticed that the gents who flirted with me were online likely hunting for other mates, I went into a tailspin. A few years later, in 2007, after another brief and unsuccessful stint online, I realized that Internet dating intensified my addiction, and I vowed to stay away.

A week after my last conversation with Vernie, on Fat Tuesday, sitting in the New Orleans airport en route to Phoenix, I knew I needed to repent. It was Lent. Time to fast from Jim and the temptation to paw and be pawed. Time to recalibrate to friends only. This time I really meant it. My three-month carnal lusty life, my drunken stupor of love fun, was over. I told myself to straighten up and get refocused on work, and I reconnected with friends I had ignored while I flitted. I needed to pull myself back into orbit and reanchor my spirit with my secure self again.

Along with the repentance came more confidence: I didn't need to respond to every man who showed me attention. I didn't need to use men as my only measure of self-worth. And, in repeatedly floundering with the wrong men, how could I possibly attract the right one? I knew I was sending mixed signals to the universe, but I didn't know why. Or how to stop. I was very clear on the qualities I was seeking in my life partner, yet again and again I got off center. It was clear that I wasn't clear at all. I didn't say, "You're not in my league. You're nowhere near what I'm seeking." Of course I didn't. I didn't tell them their kissing was horrible or that their silence and dark moods were troubling or that I'm not attracted to insecure, balding men. I certainly did not. In fact, I did just the opposite. I went to his condo, all tan and beige, with two aging cats and a broken toilet, or I drove an hour to his waterfront condo and submitted to an after-dinner grope all to satisfy my hunger for male attention—which was never satisfied. I'd feel remorse, and go right back in and grab some more.

9
Mr. Peace Corps

While my executive coaching firm, in its eighth year in 2003, was burgeoning, I was searching for something more, a higher purpose. I'd always known that coaching corporate leaders was not the end game for me. I wanted to have a greater humanitarian impact, to help those who didn't have the means to help themselves, especially the homeless, hungry, and lonely elderly with whom I'd been volunteering for fifteen years. Early that spring, I considered a two-week summer volunteer trip in Russia to visit forgotten seniors in dilapidated post–World War II housing complexes. I'd recently drawn up a plan for Executive Angels, a nonprofit outgrowth of my coaching firm that would match corporate leaders with life-changing global volunteer stints. Going to Russia for the summer was my first foray into global "angeling." I needed to experience firsthand what I had conceived. While my volunteer work had always been a solo act, my grand vision, the vision that was superglued to my brain, was to travel the globe with my life partner to serve the world's needy.

While vowing to keep my hands off Jim and sending my last e-mail to Vernie, photos of James—a Peace Corps alum and a world traveler, wearing a jaunty beret and smiling in front of Saint Basil's Cathedral in Moscow, Stonehenge, and the Alps—enticed me on Match.com. A fellow adventurer! Humanitarian kin! Peace Corps! A perfect match!

I cast an introductory note his way, flattering him with "you are handsome" and "an intriguing renaissance man" bait. He bit immediately. Over the next two weeks, we e-mailed back and forth, divulging our basic career, family, and geographic coordinates. His responses were brief, polite, and formal—which only made me try harder to be complimentary, clever, and flirty.

Our first date was on a gorgeous spring Saturday afternoon in downtown Saint Petersburg, the halfway point between his Bradenton home and my Clearwater Beach cottage. We met for lunch on the patio of a popular British colonial tavern, The Moon Under Water, overlooking shimmering Tampa Bay. James was forty-eight and attractive in a clean-cut, rugged way. He had been born in Britain, raised in Seattle, and schooled in Denver and had worked in urban planning in Alaska and, for the previous seventeen years, in various cities and counties throughout Florida.

Sitting across from one another at a tiny table, we dove right into a topic we'd discussed many times over e-mail—travel. His eyes never met mine. When he responded to my questions, he looked six inches above my eyes, seemingly at some point on the bay—the entire lunch. I thought it was nerves, shyness. It did not occur to me that James's inability to look me in the eye on our first date might be another clue: I don't want you to see the real me. I won't let you see the real me. Was he emotionally distant? Should I have run for the hills? Not a chance, not me. He was intelligent and charming, and had amazingly diverse interests. For starters, he spoke Latvian, was learning Russian, and was an expert in Louis XIV furniture. Besides, I had already cast him as the leading man in my global humanitarian dream.

After lunch, we strolled adjacent Straub Park under a canopy of old-growth banyan trees and shared our respective relationship histories.

"I've never been married," he said. He stopped walking, waiting for my reaction. "That's pretty much been a deal breaker when I've told other women on the first date."

"Well, I can see how it would be hard to settle down with you traveling and moving every few years," I said. "You've had other priorities. I can understand why you haven't found the right woman yet." His fear of intimacy, the fear of commitment that his other dates surely sniffed out on date one, completely eluded me.

"I'd love to take you out again," he said, his voice more upbeat, animated. "Would you be interested in coming down my way next Saturday?"

"Sounds like fun. I'd love to."

My car sailed home. I was buoyant with the promise of new love, singing Earth, Wind and Fire's "Got to Get You into My Life" at the top of my lungs, certain that I already had.

An hour south, James's place was a modest two-bedroom condo in a nondescript beige, early-'80s building overlooking the Manatee River. He met me in the parking lot with a polite hug and escorted me upstairs for a quick tour of his bachelor pad, which turned out to be decorated in mid-1930s grandmother. His tiny apartment walls were checkered floor to ceiling with faded frames of British military needlepoint. He led me to one of his prized samplers, an intricate embroidery of a soldier hoisting the Union Jack with the words FREEDOM, JUSTICE, AND PEACE stitched into the worn muslin.

"I've never seen anything like this before," I asked. "Where did you find these?"

"I've always been interested in British military history and started collecting them five years ago," he said. "I look at each one of these as sort of a piece of social history. See how this soldier commemorated his experience of World War I?"

I scanned the room for more artifacts. Lace doilies adorned the couch and easy chair. A passel of antique pewter drinking mugs crowded the top of the refrigerator and nook shelves.

"Wow, you've amassed quite a museum," I said.

"Wait until I show you the antique bedpan I picked up when I was at the Portobello Road Market last month."

I was momentarily concerned, but that was instantly overruled by my fascination. I'd never been with a man who cared for such things. I loved that he had such eclectic interests. All I saw was potential.

We took a short drive to Sarasota, where we toured the stunning 1926 Ringling Mansion, now a world-class art museum on sixty-six sweeping acres of pristine Sarasota Bay. Afterward, we relaxed with a glass of merlot in cruise-style steamer chaises on the Spanish-tiled terrace fronting the twinkling water and slowly melting sun. More red wine and succulent sauteed shrimp followed at a popular Gulf-front bistro on nearby Anna Maria Island. As the hours rolled by, I was becoming more enchanted with this man. *What a planner! What a romantic!* I thought as we drove back to his condo.

It was late. Time for me to head home to Clearwater. I collected my purse, ready to say good night, when James pulled me toward him in a tender embrace and kissed me passionately. When I came up for air, I couldn't move my feet. I didn't want to go; I was transfixed, magnetized by this man and his romantic touch. It had been two years, a lifetime, since I'd had sex with Byron, and James's kisses were elixir.

I was breathless but somehow managed to blurt an awkward attempt to compliment him. "I am not a slut," I said. "But I have been with many men. You, James, by far are the best kisser ever."

"Couch. Sit. Now," he uttered, clearly undone a little himself, as he motioned me to the couch, where we made out for another hour.

It was midnight, too late to make the drive home, so he set me up in the guest room, where I attempted to sleep. After he awoke at eight and made a pot of coffee, we lay in his bed clothed and made out for several hours before I had to race to get dressed to make a noon lunch back in Clearwater.

The next day James sent a thank-you e-mail: "Wow!!! Thank you for the weekend! You are a rare women. The combination of intelligence, wit, outgoing, care, and downright sexy!"

That was it. I was hooked. He was fun, attractive, bright, inspiring, calm, peaceful, and the best kisser and, I believed, the best potential lover I'd ever had. How would I keep it in perspective? I knew my pattern: the deeper we connected physically, the more emotionally volatile and attached I got. I thought I could curb my enthusiasm by telling myself to enjoy the experience of getting to know James slowly, the old-fashioned way. No frenetic rush, no expectations, no desperateness. How fun it would be to be courted—to not get sidetracked or seduced by the romance. I still did not realize the depth of my neediness, my addiction. I know now that I was doing my version of an alcoholic's bargaining—I'm just going to have one drink, and then I'll go home. Six drinks later and unable to make it to the car.

One kiss and I'm a goner. Starting up always gave me Herculean energy. Anticipating the next interlude was my drug.

The next weekend he was coming to my house for the first time. I thought I could keep it all under control, but true to form, I was nearly manic with domesticity. Deep cleaning, potting new flowers for the deck, ordering a rug for the office, stocking my wine bar, baking banana bread. It was the surge, the hormone zip I got anticipating and staging my next romantic act.

· ·

We had been seeing each other for a month, my typical milestone for going to the next base with a man—making love. There we were on a Saturday night facing one another on his living room couch when I pulled out the list of the values and goals I believed we needed to be aligned on before I got more deeply involved. As if I were at a board meeting, I presented my case: spiritual compatibility was crucial, as was agreeing on how much "we" time we desired—I did not want a long-distance relationship. I was always looking for a guarantee, something I didn't realize then. A way to mitigate risk, protect myself from eventual pain. The previous weekend, James had mentioned how attracted he was to my independence, the fact that we wanted but didn't need each other. I had to probe more. And communication— the ability to talk openly with each other about how we were feeling, when something was working, when something was not—was para- mount for me. James was reserved, quiet, a thinker, uncomfortable sharing his feelings. It was only a matter of a few weeks when I noticed that he rarely complimented me or expressed appreciation to me.

He looked at me thoughtfully and responded with care to my list. He wasn't religious, not especially spiritual, but he said he was open for discussions about it. He was accepting of my beliefs and offered to go to services with me. Check. The being needy–versus–needing someone part was an easy one. He clarified before I even asked the question. He wouldn't be in a relationship if he didn't need me for certain things. Check. But intimacy and communicating deeply were areas that James recognized might be deal breakers.

"We have some differences there. We're at the opposite ends of the scale when it comes to expressing feelings," he said. "I will try to be better." I was sure that if I respected our differences, and not demand he be a certain way, he would come along. I knew he was able to communicate how he felt honestly and openly—I'd heard him several times—but only when I initiated and pried. He could change. We plowed ahead.

Our weekends together were wonderful adventures, as James took the lead, applying his urban-planning expertise, researching places for us to explore together. We loved traveling the back roads of old Florida, where hundreds of acres of citrus groves and cattle ranches still stood, gorging on fresh grouper ceviche at a ramshackle shack in the sleepy fishing village of Cortez, and strolling the grounds at the antebellum Gamble mansion and sugar plantation. He was in his element orchestrating and packing wine, pâté, chocolate, and candles for our first overnight getaway at the Herlong Mansion in historic Micanopy, Florida, where we went antiquing, toured author Marjorie Kinnan Rawlings's humble wood-frame home, and sampled traditional frog legs, piles of crawfish, and turtle—in these parts, they are referred to as cooters—at The Yearling restaurant. When Sunday nights rolled around and it was time to drive home, I pinched myself. I was so happy.

James's kisses and caresses drove me crazy. I could not keep my hands off him. Every time we geared up for intercourse, my hunger for him was excruciating. But he would turn quiet, his face twisted in disappointment, his penis drooping.

"It's just nerves," he said. It had been a year since he had been with a woman. "Be patient with me."

"Of course," I replied.

At the end of month two and with no improvement, I asked, "Have you considered the possibility of erectile dysfunction?"

"I'm too young." He was convinced it was just a matter of time with us. He'd be fine in another few weeks; he was certain.

"Why not at least see your doctor?"

He shook his head with an emphatic no.

I gently brought it up again a few weeks later, and this time he agreed to make a doctor's appointment. The next weekend he raced from his car to my front door with a smile and a bottle of blue pills, heading to the bedroom to test their effectiveness. They worked. He worked. He was reborn. Fixing James, step one: complete. Successful.

James was my latest rehab project, and there was more work to be done. What I was also experiencing—one of the most common components of my version of love addiction—was a sort of codependency on steroids: when an addict becomes preoccupied with excessive caretaking (i.e., "fixing" the other), while completely losing sight of her own needs. Codependent Love Addicts try desperately to hold on to the people they are addicted to by using codependent behavior, according to Love Addicts Anonymous. "This includes enabling, rescuing, caretaking, passive-aggressive controlling, and accepting neglect or abuse. In general, CLAs will do anything to "take care" of their partners in the hope that they will not leave—or that someday they will reciprocate."

For a few weeks James had been complaining about his aching back. He walked with a tilt. Enjoying an alfresco breakfast on Anna Maria Island on a bright Sunday morning, the calm turquoise Gulf just steps away, I went through the list of usual culprits: A twisted muscle from overexertion? Did you lift something too heavy while refurbishing your condo? Too much stress from the latest battle at the county?

"How old is your mattress?" I asked.

"Old," he said.

Over Memorial Day weekend, we shopped for mattresses, bouncing on extra firms. His new mattress was delivered, and instantly he was pain-free. Fixing James, step two: complete. Successful.

June, soaring into the nineties already, was pool and beach time. Fair-skinned James had a smidgen of light-brown hair on his chest, arms, and legs but a thick carpet of bearlike black fur on his back. Contorting his head in the vanity mirror, he struggled to shave the pelt, leaving a prickly stubble.

"Have you ever had a back wax?" I asked.

His face winced in pain. "Never."

That Saturday after a tense thirty-minute wax at my Vietnamese salon back in Clearwater, he was delighted with his hairless, baby-soft back.

"I feel ten pounds lighter," he said.

Fixing James, step three: complete. Successful.

Insatiable

By month three his voice and e-mail messages had become more businesslike and void of the tenderness I required. Actually, they'd been perfunctory right from the start, but I'd just excused it. Now my translation was: he doesn't want to be with me. I craved his attention and adoration all the time. Not just between the sheets. Eventually, our regular evening calls felt like a download of the AP news service: a simple reporting of the day's events. He was far more comfortable discussing my central AC issues, his search for new living room carpet, refinancing rates, the quality of toilet paper in Russia, and the latest hiccup at work than he was discussing "us."

"My needs aren't being met," I told him. "It feels like we have a business partnership." I knew James was British, reserved, uneasy expressing emotions—he had said as much. And although our physical intimacy had vastly improved since the blue pills, he seemed stingier with compliments and praise. I needed to know he cared, that I was appreciated. I didn't think I was asking for much: a quick e-mail during the day to say I'm thinking about you; an occasional "You look wonderful tonight." The more he withheld, the hungrier I got. "You should already know I care for you," he said, "that I want to be with you." But I didn't. I needed acknowledgment, proof—constantly. Show me, tell me you love me. Where I know now I was justified was in wanting more from him—he really did give me very little to work with, just as he admitted he had with other women in the past. Where I went overboard, however, was in not knowing when to stop wrestling acknowledgment and affection out of him, rather than realizing I would never get what I was starving for from him.

After four months together, I had plummeted from bafflement to desperation. I smothered him in endearments, hoping I could teach him how it was done. I told him he was sexy and gorgeous, constantly. He just rolled his eyes. But occasionally he threw me a bone. "Did I tell you how much I enjoy being with you?" I asked.

"Not as much as I with you," he said. And with that, magically, I'd be back on cloud nine—at least for a few days.

What stood out most about my time with James was that in the spaces between my most euphoric and most desperate moments in our relationship, I began to see glimpses of another, more balanced perspective on the situation. Though I couldn't always recognize it, I

128

was already in the midst of my healing journey, continuing to shape-shift my foundation and gradually reprogram my old belief patterns, reorienting from unworthy to valuable; from focusing on the bad to seeing what was good; from a lens of suffering to deep gratitude; from being 24/7 self-critical to acknowledging my strengths; and from being resistant and fearful to open and trusting. I was shedding my romanticized notions, the little-girl ideals about how men are sup-posed to rescue me. I was releasing what my coach Meryl called my "security complex." I *was* making progress. I was more self-aware. I was showing evidence of growth.

However, even though on paper, in my journal day after day, I could appear healthy and lucid about my "issues" and have a clear strategy to avoid and overcome my obsessive/addictive behaviors once and for all, my reality was still another story. Despite the progress I had made, I was very much in a two-steps-forward, one-step-back mode. No matter how much I "prepped" and coached myself about what *not* to do, I continued to put too much futile effort into building a lasting relationship fortress out of a pile of quicksand. I continued to exhibit most of the classic love addiction symptoms, and I still did not grasp why I was so greedy. Why did I need, need, need so much recognition and validation? I cringe now thinking of how needy I was—expecting him to make me feel more lovable. Back then, the concept of self-love was foreign to me. I thought loving myself meant going to the spa for a pedicure, buying a new pair of shoes, or getting together with girlfriends for a glass of wine. I didn't understand how mean I was to myself. How I rejected myself by being so critical and unforgiv-ing. I didn't realize that my addiction, any addiction, is a misguided search for self-love, a form of self-rejection. I was unable to accept compliments and praise, although I longed for them. When a friend or family member asked how I was, I'd immediately volley the atten-tion back with an "Oh, we'll get to that. How are you?" I hadn't learned how to be kind and gentle and nurturing, to be a loving mother to myself. I didn't yet know the difference between wanting and needing emotional support and how I was making James responsible for my feelings. I had no idea I was abandoning myself at every turn, instead expecting a man to love and fix me. Had I been doing this my entire life? Delegating the responsibility that was only mine? Had I ever held myself accountable for my happiness? At some subterranean level, probably because I had read it in countless spiritual books—I knew that I had to love myself first before I could truly love another. But I simply did not know how to love.

Looking back, the magnitude of my dependency on James, on all the men I was with, was astonishing. Equally dismaying was how rapidly I transformed my persona. After the first month, the independent, confident, free-spirited woman who initially captivated them transmuted into a grabby, weak, needy whiner. When I read *The Cinderella Complex* a few years later, I saw for the first time who I was in every single relationship: a self-assured, successful upbeat woman with an immense unconscious fear of independence and a desire to be taken care of by others. Bait and switch. I had no idea that's what I was doing.

Lying on my oversized red couch on a Friday night, I cried out in despair. I had not talked with James for four days. He was immersed in moving to a new condo and had little time for a quick hello call, which was incomprehensible to me. I felt sick, anxious, suffering withdrawal, my brain racing with worst-case scenarios. So many tears I'd cried in desperation—terrified of being abandoned. The briefest separation triggered perceptions and misperceptions, expectations of abandonment and lost love. And there I was that Friday. *Why do I feel imprisoned by my behaviors and thoughts, so unbelievably constricted in pain, hurt, and sorrow? How can someone treat me so badly?* It was the exact same place I always found myself in with a man—realizing months later that the only person treating me badly was me.

With the precision of a forensic auditor, for three months I had been inventorying every lack of a phone call, every silent moment, every time he ignored one of my greeting cards or phone calls. Every conversation was dissected. Every perceived slight was tallied. Every moment was focused on what was going wrong and how I could I fix it. FBI-like, I scoured our dwindling relationship landscape, searching for another clue that he was slipping away. Another piece of evidence that he didn't want me anymore. Everything pointed to "getting rid of Shary."

I seemed to expect hurt and rejection even when there was no apparent reason for such anxiety. The wounds from feeling neglected by my parents were still gaping, oozing. Who knew that because I was never able to fix my parents, make them the warm and loving nurturers I longed for, I unconsciously kept inviting familiar emotionally unavailable men into my life? At a deeply invisible level, I honestly believed I was going to change the man—this time. *I know I can change you by loving you so much.* I had radar for those men who would replicate the struggle I had with my parents, in which I strived endlessly to be good enough, quiet enough, worried enough, and helpful enough to win their love.

The next morning I finally reached James on his new cell phone. He didn't want to talk. He was busy unpacking a mountain of boxes. "I feel like you're shutting me out," I said.

"It has nothing to do with you," he said. "Just let me get through this awful move." Somehow I managed to lighten up by telling him he had sent me a bunch of new contact numbers and that none of them functioned. "What a great way to avoid people," I said. He laughed. And there it was. That was all I needed. I could breathe again. We were all better. That night he left me a message while I was walking on the beach: "I hope you understand my idiosyncrasies."

Idiosyncrasy?! To me it was huge to go into a hole, to shut out those who are closest to you. For him it was normal. "Perhaps that's one of my limitations." But I thought it was an isolated incident. *Moving does require immense energy. He needs his space. He'll reemerge.*

· ·

In early July, the night before I was to leave for Russia, James and I had a reunion at my place. Between his packing and moving and traveling, we had not seen each other for three weeks. He walked into my front door, beaming like Santa, loaded with birthday gifts, mostly practical yet much-needed supplies for my trip: a pocket flashlight, a Russian dictionary, a travel journal. It was glorious to be in his arms again, to hold and kiss him. He was attentive and loving, and I felt wanted, desired, and revitalized. Brought back to life. All my trauma and sadness from the prior three weeks obliterated.

When I returned from Russia in early August, after another three weeks away from one another, all I felt was gratitude when I fell into his arms at the airport. This man fascinated me to no end. I was in love with him, and I was scared as hell that he would leave at any moment. But in *that* moment, that weekend, I had him all to myself, as we were sequestered at my beach cottage the entire rainy weekend. We holed up in bed and made love and talked, ordered Greek salads for lunch, went back to bed, ordered a Greek pizza for dinner, watched a little TV, read, and then went back to bed. It was the bliss I dreamed of, what I lived for: no distractions, no schedule, my man's full attention and ardor in my cozy lair.

Yet in early September, after another anguishing dry spell of not seeing or talking to him, I again brought up our potential deal breaker, his ability to verbalize his care and affection for me more openly. In his mind he had improved; he said complimentary things to me more frequently. But I knew that 90 percent of the time, it was in response to adulation I had initiated: "Do you know how much I adore you?"

"Not as much as I do you."

But it was more than the communication. He had been distancing himself for a while. And once again, fearing the familiar—abandonment—I put on my Savior Shary cape and went right to desperation mode, fixing, rescuing. I read relationship and marriage books and web sites. I prepared an elaborate new strategy to improve our communications.

I spent hours drafting the "IMPROVEMENT PLAN," a three-page memo about the characteristics of a conscious partnership, explaining how our respective old tapes were getting in the way and throwing in psychological assessment data from my coaching work. Not once did it occur to me that over and over again, I kept sending the same message: you are unable to meet my needs. You are inadequate.

I was certain we were meant to be. We were just overworked and stressed and needed a weekend getaway to restore ourselves. I arranged for a romantic getaway at the Shamrock Inn in Weirsdale, Florida, and sent teasing, suggestive, flirty e-mails days prior about an erotic bubble bath and a doctor's order for a full-body massage. I packed his favorite wine, new seductive lingerie, and a bottle of champagne. Saturday night in Weirsdale, while he was taking a late swim, I prepared a foamy whirlpool bath with luxurious bubbles, a chilled bottle of champagne on the side, lights dimmed, candles glowing, and me enveloped with frothy bubbles wearing my most beguiling face.

He walked in, looked and me, went to the bedroom, and turned the TV on.

"I've got something special for you," I said.

"I'll be there in a minute," he said.

He stayed glued to the TV.

Thank God, we were staying just one night, I thought, suddenly regretting launching another one of my flimsy "relationship restoration" schemes. I dried off, temporarily shelved my disappointment and joined him in bed for a chaste evening of television and making fun of our Irish Blarney room's green tartan wallpaper and jumble of leprechaun doodads.

Sure, there had been signs that he was disengaging, but I still wasn't ready to accept them. I was *never* ready to accept that fate. It only made me dig my heels in deeper. I was hanging by a thread, unknowingly panicking at the prospect of being alone again. There *had* to be a way to get us back on track.

On our drive home, I began devising my newest action plan, silently mapping out my top ten to-dos:

1. Know that God loves me and will never let me down nor leave me.
2. Embrace and appreciate James, all of James.
3. Know that I love James just as he is.
4. Just know that James loves me.
5. Listen to James thoroughly.
6. Be patient, listen intently to each word he says.
7. Give him time to think.
8. Believe and know that this is good and right.
9. Respect James in every way.
10. Know that James is my best ally.

The intensity of my self-deception—that I needed only to try harder—seems staggering to me now, but back then I was still defaulting to my self-blaming, self-effacing behaviors. I see the person I was then as yearning to be fully realized but trapped in a half-formed state of her own making.

A week after our B&B weekend, I woke James on Sunday morning, smothering him with kisses. I needed to feel close to him again and longed to make love. The tender moments, when we were connecting, were precious, rare. After, we went into town for brunch. He was remote, preoccupied—about what I didn't know. He would never tell me. When we returned, he plopped down in his easy chair and hid behind the newspaper. I thought we had plans that afternoon. "What do you want to do?" I asked. "Do you want me to leave?"

He didn't answer me directly. He wanted to read the paper, he said, and to spend a few hours researching real estate.

Suddenly, in a moment of crystal clarity, the seven-month fog of denial finally lifted. It hit me like an icy shower that he had been pushing me away for weeks, months. We'd been inching along trying to resuscitate us. Actually, I'd done all the resuscitating while he'd been a passive observer—almost as if he was waiting for me to drop the ball. It dropped.

"This is not working," I said, placing my overnight bag by the front door.

He was silent.

"How do you see us moving forward?" I asked.

Silence. He studied the worn beige carpet under his feet.

I was depleted. Tired of managing, fueling, fixing, pushing, hoping for more love. It was not there to give. Not as much as I wanted. It was an impossible demand. An impossible love.

He was mute. He wouldn't look at me. Cold. Shades of John, Patrick, Byron. Unable to face me.

I drove home feeling recharged, lighter, free of a burden I didn't realize I was carrying, proud that I had initiated something I should have done months before. The next morning I awoke early and energized, mapping my own self-improvement plan. Another pattern after breakups. I was suddenly able to see how I'd neglected myself, my friendships, family, and interests. After a breakup is when I started taking care of me, having put my best self on hold while I was in the relationship. In a flash I had my weekend and Saturday night calendar filled for the next six to eight weeks, through the holidays. I called about golf lessons; I'd put them off for months. I was ready to start volunteering at the homeless shelter again. I was right back where I had started.

10
Firsts

History refers to the 1970s, my high school and college years, as tumultuous times. They were. The deadly and divisive Vietnam War still raged. Antiwar demonstrations, including those at Kent State, where four students were gunned down, sparked across the country, while Watergate and mistrust in government, two oil crises, and severe inflation flared.

Turbulent is also how I would describe my inner world at Archbishop Alter High School. Expecting a top-notch education and discipline, in a school where nuns and priests still wore long flowing robes with huge rosaries dangling from their necks, where demerits were issued as readily as Vegas poker chips, and where a full curriculum of religious classes were requisite, I was befuddled and discouraged to find that half my classes were taught by coaches, not career teachers. We joked about how little we were learning. At least two or three girls in my class got pregnant, and by the time senior year came around, many of the football players were strung out on pot and 714s, a barbiturate-like sedative that they dropped like candy before games.

The highlight of every weekend was either sneaking with fake IDs into a dive bar called The Picnic, just off the University of Dayton campus, where we crowded into a smoke-hazed concrete room, drank longneck Hudepohl beers, and sucked Marlboro Lights, or hanging out at parties, where many kids passed out on couches or on the floor after overimbibing scary grain-alcohol-laced red punch that filled the bathtub or popping one too many pills. Occasionally I tagged along with some of my partier friends, and within minutes a sense of not belonging, being alone in a room full of people, came over me.

Unsurprisingly, high school also bolstered my dissatisfaction with my body. Surrounded by pretty and sophisticated cheerleaders, drill-team dancers, and assorted regular beauties, I automatically dismissed myself as unattractive, unappealing, and therefore unlovable. I didn't realize until many years later that I was hardly the only teenage girl who struggled with her body image, but I certainly felt like I was then. My lack of self-worth derived from my negative body image and from my general dissociation from my body. Well into my twenties, thirties, and forties, I sustained this distorted sense of my appearance.

I didn't make the connection back then between my unhappiness and my weight. I didn't realize that teen girls with low self-esteem and other emotional issues have a high likelihood of developing eating disorders. I found myself turning increasingly to food—particularly sugary candies and cookies, for comfort—to relieve feelings of anxiety and anger that I wasn't even aware I had. My mother, herself locked into a lifetime of bingeing and dieting, was my role model as I started my own cycle of secretly stuffing myself with sweets and then spitting them out.

After school, I grabbed packages of Ho Hos and a cold can of Tab and hid in my room, poring over *Teen* magazine, watching TV, and concocting dreamy scenarios with kindly older gentlemen like variety show hosts Mike Douglas and Merv Griffin. I was in love with Merv Griffin. And Paul Lynde from *Bewitched* and *Hollywood Squares*. In my teens and twenties, I imagined television and movie stars noticing me and falling in love. I was convinced that Michael Keaton and I were a match ordained by heaven after reading an interview with him in *Cosmopolitan* about the type of woman he was looking for. *That's me!* I thought. Oh, how convinced I was. I unknowingly relied more and more on my imagination to stir up happy feelings to soothe myself, to make my otherwise dismal life bearable. I now realize that my imagination and later my actual love life were the places I'd go to enliven my emotional life, to offset all my negative feelings. I hoped and wished and waited for and fantasized about love while having absolutely no familiarity with it.

When I wasn't watching TV, doing housework, or doing homework,

I closed my eyes and lost myself in sad songs that I played over and over again on my big, boxy record player. The Carpenters' "Rainy Days and Mondays" and Bread's "Everything I Own" solaced me for hours. And I was sure Janis Ian's "At Seventeen" had been written for me; she knew all about the anguish and hyperactive imaginations of overlooked high-school girls.

· ·

Simple embarrassments seemed to paralyze me. I looked for any excuse to avoid Wednesday PE class, when I had to wear school-supplied, gold, nylon shorts that exposed my thick, dimply thighs, normally camouflaged under my uniform skirt. Worse were the wheelbarrow races and seeing the dread or disgust on my partner's face, knowing she would never win because she had to push me, surely the fattest girl in the class—or so I thought—fifty yards across the gym floor. I often feigned being doubled over from a too-intense period to get out of PE.

The most innocent of comments stung me well beyond the normal grace period for such infractions. Friends from Incarnation School, the ones with long, straight hair, still called me Bubba, a name they had given me in sixth grade for my softball-sized pigtails of frizz, which they referred to as "bubbas." I laughed with them but ached inside, feeling uglier and more of an outsider by the day. When Sister Katherine, the algebra teacher, pulled me aside one early winter morning to tell me in a stern voice that my pants were too tight, unbecoming of a young lady in a Catholic school, I was horrified for being singled out. And for how I looked! That was far worse an offense than getting reprimanded for talking in class or not having completed homework. I wasn't trying to be sleazy; they were the only pants I had that fit me. But it didn't matter. For the rest of the day, I attempted to hide my back end by pulling down my regulatory maroon cardigan, but it didn't work. I became even more self-conscious and vowed never to wear pants again, despite the long stretch of frigid January temperatures I had to endure.

Others, like my mother and sister Nancy, were Teflon-like, impervious to off-hand remarks and criticism. I was amazed at how other girls and boys, disabled or fatter or zittier than I, rose above. Their backbones seemed to propel them to become determined fighters and achievers, and emboldened them with an "I'll show them" attitude. I, on the other hand, got swallowed. I didn't know how to root myself. If I imagined someone looking at me the wrong way, laughing at me, or, worse, ignoring me, I internalized it as truth, tormenting and trapping myself in a self-conscious stew of profound loneliness, melancholy, and gnawing hopelessness.

Here is one of those "I wish I knew then what I know now" lessons: teen angst is normal. Every adolescent feels insecure and anxious, worried about how he or she is seen by others. All teens compare themselves to one another. And at some point all kids feel like they don't fit in—that no one understands them. Psychologist Erik Erikson said that adolescence is when one begins to develop a stronger identity—a direction and purpose in life—and starts to gain a sense of what he or she wants to do and be. But some adolescents become more uncertain about what the future might hold for them. They are generally not goal-focused. Rather, they drift aimlessly, confused about where they might end up—that is, they have an identity crisis. That was the route I took, stuck in my own little hell of self-absorption, creating a more distorted image of myself, unable to envision a greater life. I didn't know what depression was back then. I observed my mom, who seemed perpetually unhappy and exhausted. I didn't realize that I, too, was starting to turn my unconscious rage about being neglected and rejected against myself. I was in what author and Buddhist teacher Tara Brach calls the trance of unworthiness. Trapped. Clueless about who I really was. Robotic. Go to school. Come home from school. I was obedient. Silent—until my escalating anger erupted.

One evening I lashed out at my youngest brother, Bill, when he politely requested that I not put so much mustard on the salami sandwich I was packing for his school lunch. "Do it yourself!" I yelled, throwing his sandwich across the counter, mustard splattering down the cabinets. After walking home from school another afternoon, I found the backdoor—normally opened—locked. I knocked on the door for five minutes, knowing my brother Jim was already inside. I looked in the windows, yelling for him to open the door. I could hear him laughing and taunting, "Too bad, fatty," as I bashed in the door window with my bare hand.

I see now how essential it is for teens living in their heads as much as I did to find some sort of lifeline to affirm their value—to show them they have worthwhile talents and gifts. They need someone to say, "Nonsense. You're blowing things way out of proportion. Look at all your great qualities." They need an angel, a teacher, an aunt—anyone—to say, "You is kind. You is smart. You is important," the loving words of encouragement that the character Aibileen in the movie *The Help* repeated to the little girl under her care whose mother berated her constantly.

When I turned sixteen, in the summer of 1973, Steve, a boy I had a crush on in eighth grade, asked me out on my first date. We saw each other every day at the Oakday Beach Club—such a fancy name for a giant square pool plopped near the railroad tracks on a sketchy side of town. I don't recall talking to Steve. We may have said hello in the foosball and pinball room, where he, my brothers, and other boys hung out during rest period, gulping cherry snow cones and frozen Milky Ways. But when he asked me one afternoon if I wanted to go a movie that Saturday night, I couldn't contain my excitement. I had a date! My first date! I was finally of the age my mother deemed fit for dating, and she took me shopping to pick out a new outfit for the occasion: white cotton bell bottoms and a pink Pappagallo pullover sweater. For the first time, I felt that my life might turn out okay.

When Steve opened the door of his white 1973 Impala for me, I was in heaven. Pink Floyd playing on the eight-track tape player, we drove across town to the drive-in theater to see *American Graffiti*. The romantic possibilities I had invented in my head now had the potential to unfold, but I was quiet around Steve. I didn't know how to act or what to say. He was more worldly and experienced with girls, or so I thought. I didn't want to make a mistake. When he pulled me close and put his arm around me, I felt wanted and secure for the first time—but then it was over. We had just that one date. Four weeks later, the school year started, and we went our separate ways; I was going into my junior year at Alter High, and Steve returned to Chaminade High, downtown. We had no further contact, although I longed for it, imagining how I'd run into him at church on Sundays or that he'd call me to go to the Alter–Chaminade football game with him.

My second date in four years of high school was with Kevin, a popular, thin, and freckled football player who asked me to go to homecoming my senior year. I later found out that the only reason I had a date with Kevin was because my girlfriends felt sorry for me and wanted me to have a homecoming date my final year. They had convinced Kevin to ask me out. To this day, I have no idea how they got him to agree to it. I was certain he had a girlfriend. I sat with my friend Kathy, who had a date with Kevin's best friend, Bill, on the hard, cold bleachers, our plate-sized yellow pom-pom mum corsages plastered to our coats, watching Kevin and Bill run down the field. What I didn't realize then, but should have expected, was that Kevin and several of the football players were high that night. After the game, Kevin was strung out. I don't remember him saying hello or us going to the dance. What I do recall was Bill driving with Kathy in the front seat and Kevin and me in the back. He was reclining, his eyes shut, his mouth moving, but he wasn't saying anything. We didn't exchange a word. I told them to take me home. That was senior homecoming, a date I prepared and primped for for weeks.

The summer after graduation, after I convinced my parents that I wanted to be Jacques Cousteau's assistant, my dad drove me to Florida in his white Datsun 240Z, his marine locker crammed in the hatchback, packed with first-year college necessities. The University of Tampa, a tiny school on the Hillsborough River, was my new home—nine hundred miles away from Ohio. At last, at seventeen, I was going to be on my own. Free! Free of being the oldest of six, the obedient little mother.

The University of Tampa was a tiny school, with just 700 students, and we incoming freshmen numbered no more than 150 students from all over the country. I loved that everyone was in the same boat, getting to know one another, unlike the long-held friendships from high school that were difficult to penetrate. Conversations and friendships were easy, and for the first time, when boys came up to me to talk, I didn't shy away.

Florida was heavenly. And I became a hellion. I lay out in the sun on the banks of the river, skipped classes, and mooched rides to the beach. I smoked my first cigarette, sipped my first banana daiquiri, and inhaled my first joint. I had another first: my first D, in freshman biology. My childhood fantasy to sail the seas with Jacques was obliterated. The truth was revealed: I hated rigid, methodical science. I was enchanted with words and writing. Was it the sunshine, the salt water, the chance to start a new life far from those who knew the old me? Carrying the usual extra twenty pounds, with my hair in a large Afro and my skin dark brown from a full summer of tanning, I was still hyper-self-conscious. But in Florida I was happier, more confident, and carefree. I sensed the possibility of a rebirth. I was in love with Eric, a handsome Irish guy with a wild and tough streak from Miami. A cigarette always hanging off his lips and a head of light-brown, sun-streaked, curly hair, he was the sexiest boy-man I'd ever known, and God, how I wanted him to like me. He had a girlfriend back home; her name came up now and then, and he showed me a picture of her once. A dark-haired, dark-eyed beauty.

Although Eric was never interested in me romantically, we became pals. One night I was the designated driver of his white Malibu, but I ended up high, as he and I passed a joint back and forth while I drove seventy miles per hour on the downtown freeway—just another testament to the fact that I would do anything for love.

The boy who *was* interested in me was Mike (Big Red), a strapping, six foot three, redheaded teacher's assistant and ROTC nut on scholarship. Obsessed with his dream of being an officer and airborne, parachuting out of planes and helicopters in war zones with his troops, he turned out to be a buddy and an occasional date but was too straitlaced and serious for me to consider as a boyfriend. The semiwild boys like Eric, who smoked and cussed and had a what-the-hell attitude, were the ones I thought were sexy. But Mike was apparently enamored with me and for a nineteen-year-old was a thoughtful romantic. He bowed upon delivering a single red rose to me one afternoon in my dormitory lobby. And after a fancy dinner celebrating the end of the school year, I opened a carefully wrapped blue box to find a lovely silver necklace and locket. Up to that point, we hadn't been especially affectionate—only chaste hugs and kisses on the cheek. Yet after dinner and a late stroll on campus, there we were in my saggy single bed, smashed against the grimy dorm-room wall, naked. I think I was more curious about sex than wanting Mike to be my first lover. I was shaking, so scared that I was going to bleed to death or do something wrong. I barely moved. It was unremarkable. Neither of us said much afterward.

Everyone remembers the first time they had sex, don't they? I recall very little of that night except the dorm room. Did he try to kiss me after dinner? Is it simply a faded memory or was I emotionally numb? Was I unable to deal with the overwhelming emotions of having sex for the first time? I'd been dreaming about my first lover for how many years, yet I can't remember how I felt or what was said?

What I know now about that night is that it did not unfold as I had romanticized. No night ever could. My longing for love was my lifeblood—far more important than actually *having* it. There was no way Mike or any mere mortal could ever deliver upon that illusion. My addiction to romance and love became only more deep-rooted that night.

11
The Good Guy #2

One early morning at the gym three months after my breakup with James, I was struggling on the bicep-curl machine when Chris walked over and stood by me.

"Hi", he said, looking apprehensive. "Would you like to have lunch next Friday?"

It was eerie how much he looked like Doug. Chris seemed sweet-tempered, patient, and thoughtful and a lot like I imagined Doug would look if he were twenty years older.

I later found out that he asked me out the day after his divorce was finalized. Apparently, he had been waiting months to make his move. I wasn't attracted to Chris. I just knew him as someone to have a quick friendly chat with at the gym.

"I've got client meetings all day Friday," I said. But I reluctantly agreed to meet him for coffee the following week.

Sitting in a hard, straight-backed chair at Starbucks on a chilly early-December Sunday afternoon, I was unenthusiastic, brusque. I acted like I had better things to do on a Sunday. When he asked me what I enjoyed doing in my spare time, I babbled about being a dabbler.

"I love trying so many things," I said. "I've taken belly-dancing, sushi-making, and windsurfing lessons. But I never stick with any of them long enough to get good. I'm so disappointed in myself."

"Sounds like you are a passionate woman. You have the unique ability to pursue a lot of possibilities," he reassured me. He leaned back in his chair and looked at me thoughtfully. Steaming mug in his hand, he looked like a university professor. "That's not a negative at all. It's a gift."

Instantly, his kindness and sincerity softened me. I relaxed my stiff businesslike posture and looked at him with new eyes. Nearly nine years older than I, fifty-five, silver haired and bespectacled, Chris was grounded, encouraging, and insightful in a gentle way. *This man is warmhearted, a good soul. He'll take care of me,* I unconsciously registered, noting the homines of his red plaid flannel shirt.

It turned out that his and Doug's birthdays were a day apart, which I took as some sort of sign. I had asked for an older Doug, hadn't I? He was the man with whom I'd had my longest relationship—six years. And here he was again. It was true that I hadn't been attracted to Doug in the beginning, either, but I had grown to love him. And from the intense way Chris was looking at me now, I knew he was smitten. Sharklike, I unknowingly sensed bounty—a virgin source of perpetual attention. I wouldn't have to be obsessive. He'd give me no reason to doubt.

Although I felt no spark with Chris, I knew he'd be a good friend— or, at the very least, a kayaking buddy. We finished our coffee and agreed to meet the following Sunday afternoon at the beach for a hot toddy to celebrate the holiday season.

During the next month, Chris and I had a kayak outing and went to a spinning class. Before long he was tagging along to an art gallery opening and offering to help me shop for a new bike. I resumed my pattern: he became my friend and my lover. But in short order I learned that his life was potholed with problems. Fresh out of a twenty-two-year marriage with a demeaning wife, Chris had a derailed career, little money, zero confidence, a car on its last legs, and a laundry list of health issues, including untreated ADHD. Jackpot: my kind of guy.

At the time, I believed I was in Chris's life to help him transition from a long miserable marriage to a fresh life filled with possibility. I had such empathy for this man who'd had a series of unlucky breaks. And I saw so much untapped talent and good in him. Plus, this is what

I did every day as an executive coach. I helped leaders and executives realize more of their potential. I could help him. He simply needed a month or two to get settled, financially and emotionally, from his divorce. He needed a career path to fuel his strengths.

I also knew that I'd been blessed in my life and thought that this was the right time to pay back the unconditional love Doug had shown me. I had sucked the life out of Doug. Now it was time for me to repay. Oh, the fibs I told myself. It was uncanny how I believed it was my God-given duty to help this man, to fix him. He didn't ask for my help, but I assumed the savior role nevertheless: *Let me be the one to carry the weight of helping Chris see the Promised Land. Please.*

Years later it became clear that Robin Norwood, author of one of my love addiction bibles, *Women Who Love Too Much,* was talking about me when she wrote, "Almost nothing is too much trouble, takes too much time, or is too expensive if it will 'help' the man you are involved with."

While I was emphatically parroting my same old tune—I want to be friends; I'm not looking for anything serious—from the other side of my mouth I found myself inviting him over on a Saturday night for Thai carryout and a bottle of cabernet.

"I'd been wondering why you've been keeping your distance," Chris said between bites of pad Thai. "I've been wanting to hold your hand, put my arm around you, but you seemed a little standoffish."

"You just got divorced," I said. "I'm the first woman you've dated in twenty-two years. You're vulnerable. You need your space. I don't want to be the rebound girl."

"This is not a horse race. We can take our time," Chris said. "But I don't want to be just your friend. I want more."

After dinner we refilled our wine glasses and relaxed on my comfy couch for several hours. He told me he trusted me already, something he hadn't ever felt in his marriage. We talked about God—he was a devout Catholic—and spirituality, a whole part of me left unexpressed in my recent relationships with James and Byron. It was emancipating.

I looked at him with his thick head of silver hair and blue eyes, wearing a blue denim shirt, and thought how attractive he really was.

I took a couple of sips of wine and lay back to perch my legs on the couch. I felt his warm hands massage my feet, and I purred.

But then I thought, *Oh shit. What happened to your friends-only rule Shary?* And the next moment I smiled to myself, thinking how this man was honest, wise, insightful, sage, quiet, strong, vulnerable, open, not needy, not desperate, straightforward. He admitted that things were awkward when they were. I liked that a lot. I was attracted to that more than anything.

In month two, he told me I was a significant part of his life. "I'm trying to control my hunger for you," he said. "You are too important to me to mess things up." He seemed so certain. It scared me. And thrilled me. I liked being with someone who was more certain about me than I was.

In bed for the first time, he shocked me by how he knew how to touch me in all the right ways. Knowing his marriage had been largely sexless for years, I had expected him to be tentative and fumbling. But instead he knew. And he looked at me, *into* me, directly, for a long, long time. He saw something in my eyes, in my soul. I was afraid to ask what. I was in awe that someone who had been in my life on the periphery for all that time, someone with whom in a million years I wouldn't have dreamed of connecting, had turned out to be a terrific match. "Chris is the greatest man I've been with," I wrote in my journal. "He makes me feel safe and wanted. I feel blessed."

By month five, true to form, I was laser-focused on Chris's potential, his courageous will to re-architect his life at fifty-five. I went on a campaign to fix the things standing in his way. I found an ADHD counselor in New York City, who coached Chris over the telephone. I had his hormone levels tested by my Ohio doctor, served as an unpaid business and marketing consultant for his video production start-up, helped him shape up his home, bought him clothes, paid for our getaways, and prepared a heap of delicious meals.

One Friday I dedicated my day to leading Chris through a strategic-planning session to create a business plan for his video production start-up. Just days earlier, I had given him a copy of one of my favorite books, Dr. Seuss's *Oh, The Places You'll Go!*, with an uplifting card. I was always, always cheering, coaching. Go team go. I told myself to

stop, stop, stop. Stop caretaking. But I didn't stop. The lie kept loop-
ing. I believed we had been brought together so I could learn to put
another's needs first, to not be so selfish. But my resentment kept
silently building—*Why isn't he paying? Why doesn't he care for me like
I do for him? Why doesn't he do the things I do for him?*—and I became
increasingly angry with myself for *again* falling into the same pattern I
was adamant about avoiding: overcompensating in the giving department to receive love. I still didn't fully understand how embedded my
working belief about myself was: I had to earn love by overachieving
and rescuing others from their pain. It was fossilized, like the trilo-
bites I used to hunt for in the limestone creek beds behind our house
on Brookway Road when I was seven.

· ·

Right on cue, after six months, sex with Chris became obligatory, just
as it had with Doug. The shine of a brand-new man had worn off.
Even kissing felt forced. Yet I persevered for the cause of "us."

It struck me later how many hundreds of times over the years I
had written in my journal about Chris, James, Byron, Doug, virtually
all the men I'd been with, "Just love him, be good to him, listen to
him, he's a good man, don't give up." Well, yes. Don't be a bitch. But
I missed the entire point. Why love someone I wasn't in love with?
Why act and behave like I was in a relationship and force myself to
love, show kindness, when the entire "relationship" was a ruse, only
the drug of the moment? I convinced myself that it was some sort of
holy obligation, a work of service, to better my "lovingness" with these
gents—when the more charitable act would have been to leave them
the fuck alone in the first place.

Doug had been right. He had told me in 1997, in our final month
together, that I needed to be with an asshole. Apparently it was true:
I was attracted to men who didn't want me. I was convinced I wasn't
good enough, so why would I bring someone into my life who thought
I was? Both Doug and Chris had attempted to show me that I *was
good* enough. But I wasn't ready to hear it. I seemed to prefer, was
accustomed to, the pain that was brought on by men: their emotional
distance, abandonment, leading me on and then backing off. Doug
and Chris gave me none of that, only steady, predictable love. No fun

in that. I had to make myself miserable. I created my own pain and suffering and added those factors to my list of addictions.

Chris and I stumbled along for eight more months. There seemed to never be a time, never a weekend, when we were free of something nagging, pulling us down. I'd fly off the handle in a second and bawl like a baby the next; my sex drive was nil. Chris was certainly trying, but his lack of a job, a purpose, and a steady income was taking a toll. Plus, I had dragged it out of him that he'd been off the new ADHD meds his doctor had put him on two weeks earlier. He'd gained weight, looked old and haggard, and we weren't having fun. I lashed out at him for not taking care of himself. Then I'd berate myself: *If I really loved him, wouldn't I care for him in a different way? I really don't know what love is.* And the endless self-diminishing loop would continue: *I'm not capable of loving the way I want to love. I'm trapped, stuck.* Most of my angst was driven by the same issue that drove Doug and me apart. I didn't like who I was with Chris. I was nagging and bitchy and tired—an exact replica of the wife he was finally free of. My issues—our issues—seemed so weighty and insurmountable that it was easier to flee. I didn't want to add a burden to Chris's huge stack.

After a little over a year together, we broke up. I needed to take a break. I needed to understand why I was not more loving with Chris—not capable of receiving his love.

I immersed myself in codependency books after my coach, Meryl, suggested that I look into the Caron Institute in Pennsylvania, an addiction facility. At the time, I discounted her suggestion. I thought codependency was something strictly associated with alcoholics. *What on earth do I have in common with alcoholics and drug addicts?* But later, when I came across an online checklist about being codependent, I checked most of the boxes. I also returned to therapy with a new counselor, Debra, in another attempt to understand why I resisted closeness and true intimacy—why I pushed love away, not only with men but with everyone. Why was there a disconnect in me when I heard compliments and words of love and appreciation from friends, family, and clients? "It's there in your head," Chris said. "You hear the words, you can read the words, but you don't feel them. You don't receive them."

Today I know that the unconscious barter of the codependent love addict—*I'll take care of you if you make me feel more lovable, safe, desired*—is rarely successful. In taking care of broken men, we fix more, obsess more, deplete ourselves more, all while avoiding our own brokenness. The artificial feelings of self-worth we get from helping others are never satisfying.

But up until I began delving more deeply into my codependent tendencies, I spent 95 percent of my time in conversation with family, friends, acquaintances, and clients talking about *them*. I loved diving in and understanding the inner workings of others. Praise and compliments rolled off my tongue with ease. I loved affirming the value I saw in each person. But when people asked me about me, I'd divert and boomerang the questions back to them. I'd always deflect a compliment. That's the way it had always been. Naturally, family and friends got accustomed to me being their private therapist, yakking on about themselves the entire time. Those were the rules—the rules that I'd established. By the time I hit my forties, I'd built up a mountain of resentment. I started noticing and asking myself: *Why am I so exhausted and hurt after talking nonstop with Ann for two hours about her life, without a breath about me?* I needed to be heard. I needed to be acknowledged and appreciated. I had set the game of life up on my terms, but the terms didn't feel good anymore. I gradually got more courageous and told my best friends and sisters that I really needed to talk about me too. I counseled clients all day. I needed to be listened to and loved, I said. I was progressing but still had a long way to go.

A month after the breakup, Chris and I got back together. It wasn't official. It just happened. The day after Valentine's Day, I agreed to meet him at the mall. He had interviews coming up, he said, and wanted my help in selecting the right business suit. What I realized after the fact was that he wanted me to see him in a suit to show me he was moving forward, was serious about launching his second career in the video-production industry. We got out of our cars in the parking lot in front of Men's Wearhouse and he stared at me with his knowing smile, moving toward me as if he were ready to kiss me. I didn't feel it. I felt only friendship. But I missed his company. I missed being wanted. And Chris seemed different. He had a new energy, a sharper focus. We drifted back together as if we'd never been apart. Chris was diligent in building new business contacts during the day and studying at night, while I desperately tried to keep my weekly therapy session amid my crowded work demands.

In our initial session, Debra used the word *trauma* to characterize my neglected childhood. I recoiled. It was the first time I had heard that word associated with my upbringing. *Trauma* sounded like a hurricane, a catastrophic event. "That's not me," I told her. But maybe it was. Maybe I'd minimized my experiences to manage the pain.

Learning to nurture and mother myself was the mission, Debra told me, something Meryl had been saying for years. After hearing me lament and sob over so many heartbreaks, Meryl would say, "You don't need fixing. Self-compassion is the only piece you're missing." At the time, I had only an inkling of what she meant. "You need to reclaim your little girl who was undermothered, underparented," Debra now said. "You have to grieve your lost childhood and rescue your little girl. You will need to learn how to start nurturing her needs, relearn how to love yourself." On the surface, it seemed easy enough. But I *do* take care of myself, I told Debra. I wasn't neglecting myself—at least in the obvious ways. But dig deeper, and you could see the evidence: I was hyper-tough on and critical of myself. I thought that was a good thing. I thought pushing and driving myself meant I would be more successful—and happy. Wrong. I knew about self-love, I coached about self-love, but I never really *got* self-love beyond taking care of myself in superficial ways. Eat well, exercise frequently, take time for me, get regular manicures, get an occasional massage—the fundamentals. But I began to understand that loving myself went far beyond that.

According to Debra, full healing would come only when I could understand how I had overlooked caring for the one who mattered most: me. Completely empty from filling everyone's cup but my own, I realized that I needed to start asking for what I wanted from others. I couldn't give and let it be about them all the time. I needed to learn to communicate that I needed support from others. I could not always be the strong, certain, I-know-everything, I-can-take-care-of-everyone oldest sister. I needed advice, support, and care too. I needed to learn to be vulnerable; asking for help was okay. Asking for support was healthy, not a weakness.

Mothering Ourselves by Evelyn Bassoff, one of the books Debra lent me, was another godsend in helping me connect the dots. "So desperate for the motherlove they missed and continue to crave," Bassoff writes, "they turn to relationships primarily to be mirrored and adored and filled up by another. Emotionally starved, they use their partners to feed their egos, but are unable to be truly supportive and loving toward their partners."

After Debra, and after I continued my grueling Theophostics spiritual counseling for another year to release more of my toxic psychic memories, I hoped I would be more open and loving to Chris. We had been together two years. But he couldn't get hold of life and move forward—at least not fast enough for me. Fits and starts toward success seemed to be part of his pattern. I had been my typical idealist self, delusional in thinking we would get through the rough patch in his life, I'd get healed, and then we'd be all better. But all he wanted—all any man wants—was for his woman to love and support him as he was. I'd loved Chris only when I could see him in a better place, with a better home, better job, better finances, better life. I couldn't accept him as he was.

In our final months, I remember saying to myself and to him, "If I cannot make it work with you, then I cannot make it work with anyone." Chris was my last shot. My God. How I limited myself. My vision of what was possible in love was realized only by what was available to me at the moment. I didn't have a greater vision for love. I was like the goldfish that swims in circles in a six-inch bowl its entire life and when put in a bathtub, the equivalent of an ocean, continues to circle in its six-inch path near the drain. Never venturing beyond.

I know now why I stayed in the relationship with Chris as long as I did. During those two years, I mostly wondered why I was staying, since it was fraught with issues. Now I have the tools to see that it was more of a healing relationship—in fact, a gift. I had lots of work to do, and Chris gave me the safe and loving haven I needed to work on myself. And I had a man who was willing, who wanted to grow and change just as much as I did.

But I had realized too late that there was no joy in being a one-woman *Extreme Makeover* episode. My overmanaging, overcritical, bossy ways—playing the all-capable, indispensable fixer—sucked the life out of me, and out of our relationship. His dependence on me emasculated him. Ultimately, we both saw that being together was too draining for us and ended our relationship amicably. It was the most peaceful breakup in my history.

Looking back on most of my relationships, I realized that by hooking up with men who needed me in some way, I held them hostage. I could take care of them on some level. I could handle the obvious stuff that I was good at: professional polishing and grooming, feeding and building romantic nests. I could do the motherly caretaking I had been practicing since I was three. So I could get what I needed from them (appreciation, unconditional love, loyalty), but I wasn't able—didn't know how or wasn't willing—to give all of my heart. No, that was too scary, too risky. The truth is, I unconsciously got involved with many weaker, less-than men so I could maintain control in order to feel more significant. I took care of fixer-uppers to feel superior. The Wizardess of Odd, I propped them up so I could prop me up. I was Sister Shary, fraudulently mixing charity and intimacy to bolster my paltry self-esteem. Sometimes I felt superior. Most of the time I felt inferior. Unlike Goldilocks, I rarely felt just right.

12
The Yogi

I was in another mini–manic phase: adrenaline, three hours of fitful sleep a night, juggling an insane all-time high of forty clients while traveling to seven cities in three months. I had a steady flow of visitors too. My mom from Ohio was staying with me for a week. Then my best friend, Kathy, was coming into town in two weeks. I also managed to find slots for an occasional date with one or two Match.com leftovers and a new friend I met walking on the beach. I was running on fumes. I had a brief respite in work coming up, and I wanted to play, be social, meet new, interesting people, laugh, and dance. I didn't realize it until I stopped to think that I had had my head down for ten months, since breaking up with Chris, with continuous work and travel. I'd been in my Bat Cave for too long. Now I could feel a new surge of autumn fun and frolic emerge—which in my case always involved a new man.

I pulled into the parking lot at Twenty-second and Gulf Boulevard in Indian Rocks Beach for the Thursday evening yoga class. It was mid-August and hot. I quickly grabbed my yoga mat from the trunk, anxious to get to the beach and feel the Gulf breeze. An old-model white Cadillac pulled into the parking space next to me. A tall, white-haired man with a Cheshire-cat grin jumped out, yoga mat and blanket in hand.

"Good evening!" he said, eyeing me up and down.

Flee. Fast. I had an immediate visceral instinct that a wily predator was stalking me. I managed a polite but brusque, "Good evening" and picked up my pace to the beach.

Savasana on the white sand, porpoises skimming by, and the instructor, Tom's, soothing voice, were just what I needed to decompress my overwrought body and mind. Tonight was potluck night, so after class I retrieved a cooler packed with shrimp mousse and a bottle of sauvignon blanc from my car and joined the forming circle, where we were to share our names and things we were grateful for.

When it got to the white-haired man, whose name turned out to be Jerry, he took to the stage, blabbing on in a self-assured manner that I read as cocky, like a morning radio DJ. He was from Chicago. In Florida for just over a year, Jerry was a retired school principal, recently divorced after twenty-seven years of marriage, and had had open heart surgery two years earlier. "It opened up my heart and transformed my life . . . my spiritual path," he shared.

Jerry appeared to be everything I now shunned: overconfident, overtalkative, overly self-important, convinced that every word he uttered was significant—the very same profile that had attracted me to my ex-husband, John, and then to Patrick a year after my divorce. But that had been twenty-three years earlier, when I was in my late twenties. Then I'd been painfully insecure, seduced by brazen and bold men, hoping that some of their mojo would seep into my sheepish pores. Now, listening to Jerry, all I saw was pomposity. A newbie on the spiritual path, Jerry seemed in awe of his own journey, as if he were the first in this universe to experience a message from God. More disquieting were the subtle hunger, desperation, and neediness lurking under his jocular walk and smile. I recognized his disguised desire for attention.

On a Sunday morning six weeks later, in the church parking lot, I saw six foot four, lean, bronzed Jerry stride toward me, looking as if he had walked off the pages of an Eddie Bauer catalog: a fit, athletic, executive type in a lavender polo shirt and khaki shorts. *He looks good,* I thought, before I could stop myself, but then quickly regained my bearings as I remembered how unpleasant I'd found his company the first time I'd met him.

"What's he doing here?" I mumbled to myself, scanning the lot for a quick getaway path. Too late.

"Good morning," he announced, his white teeth flashing. "Wow, don't you look nice."

"Thank you," I said. "I didn't know you came to Unity."

"Yes, every Sunday. I love this church. I love Leddy." Leddy was the minister.

Love. Love. Love. So much love. So much awe.

His blue eyes locked onto mine. We talked about my recent trip to Ohio to visit family and shared yoga news. He listened. Intently. Whereas I had initially experienced him as cocky and disingenuous, I now was surprised to sense sincerity, even warmth. He wanted to know more about my family.

"So, you've been coming here for a while too?" he asked.

"A year or two on and off. I always seem to be seeking."

"Me too. I'd really love to hear more about your spiritual journey. Why don't we get together for coffee or lunch sometime?"

He seemed genuine, even a bit ministerial. Maybe there was substance there after all.

"Sure," I said.

Three hours later Jerry called. I didn't answer the phone. He wanted to have dinner that night. I didn't call him back. I had a knot in my gut already. I liked being pursued, but not pressured. It was too soon for a call. Why couldn't he have waited a few days, a week? He had the exact same intensity and hunger I had detected from John and Patrick. I felt rushed and overpowered. I wanted to keep things at my pace, leisurely. Plus, *he's too old and too preachy*. Something was off, but I didn't trust myself well enough to know what. Against my better judgment, I called Jerry the next day and we set our first date.

Two weeks later, on a beautiful, seventy-five-degree, mid-October evening, I met Jerry at my favorite seaside restaurant, Guppy's. That's when I found out he was sixty-four, a few years older than I thought, and definitely hot to trot. He wasn't flirty with me; he was respectful, a gentleman. But I could tell he was one of those guys who was ultra aware of women and how they responded to him. He was hungry for a woman's attention and it showed.

He was also very attractive. He was an attentive listener, kind, and earnest in his quest for spiritual growth and transformation. I knew there had to be women lined up. Women fell in love with that kind of man every day, especially in this part of Florida, where the man-to-woman ratio is roughly one to five. Jerry had had two long-term marriages. Upon arriving in Florida, he'd landed at the Unity Church in Clearwater. He'd immediately struck up a three-month relationship, followed by a nine-month relationship—both with "Unity girls." That's how he referred to them, and now to me. Yes, he was dating one or two other women. But he didn't sound particularly attached to anyone at the moment.

"So what about you? What are you looking for?" he asked.

"I don't want the seriousness of a relationship right now," I said. "I just want to have friendships with men, keep it casual and light."

"We're in the same boat," he said. "The last thing I want is to get tied down again. I've been given a new lease on life, and I intend to live it up if you know what I mean!" He raised his glass of cabernet and arched his eyebrows, squinting in a seductive George Clooney pose.

He picked up his fork to rake the uneaten rice on his plate, seemingly in deep thought.

"Actually, the truth is, I want a woman who can take care of me."

Did he really just say that? I thought. Then I chuckled and gave him a cocky "We wouldn't work, then. I want exactly the same thing."

"But you know what they say," he said, winking. "Like attracts like. Going after the same thing in a relationship just might make it even more intriguing for us."

Despite my ever-present misgivings, Jerry seemed like the ideal tonic for my entertainment-starved self—the perfect play buddy. What I really wanted to do was go roller-skating with him. Jerry said he had been skating on the county park trails for a few months—not Rollerblading but old-fashioned roller-skating. It sounded like so much fun!

We had coffee, I thanked him for dinner, and I promised I'd reciprocate sometime soon when my schedule slowed down.

I was doing again the very thing I chastised myself for after every relationship ended: playing the man role, initiating dates, paying for dates. This one happened to be looking for a sugar mama, someone to take care of him financially. Great. I was falling back into my old pattern, the addiction that didn't have a name just yet. Later, when I began to understand I had an addiction, I found out that addictive people are typically adept at power plays. It was all about trying to stay in control at all times, to "Keep the focus outward and feel nothing inside," according to Robin Norwood.

Two weeks after our first date, I asked Jerry to join me for dinner and the Clearwater Jazz Holiday. This night was on me. I made reservations at Bobby's Bistro, a terrific restaurant on the beach, and was able to secure precious VIP tickets for the jazz fest courtesy of one of my City of Clearwater clients.

Jerry arrived at the restaurant twenty minutes late, looking flustered and complaining that the directions I had given him were wrong, wearing a pair of shorts and flip-flops. I was disappointed. It was a Saturday night. I was dressed up. We were going to be in the VIP section, not sitting on a blanket on the lawn crammed next to tens of thousands of sweaty onlookers.

"It's good to see you," I said as he slumped down in the banquette. "I'm having the Syrah. It's lovely. What would you like?" I asked, hoping to boost his spirits.

"I'm going for the hard stuff tonight," he said, motioning the waiter to our table. "A gin and tonic, with lime. Make it a double."

He slurped his escargot and shoveled the filet mignon. "This steak is fantastic. Thank God you're paying."

"Never again," I mumbled under my breath.

After a five-minute drive over the bridge to downtown Clearwater, we arrived at the festival. I immediately saw people I knew. My social butterfly took over. I said hello and hugged Melanie from the gym, and there was Martha and Craig from my class at Leadership Pinellas and the lady from Publix. I was having so much fun chatting, introducing others to Jerry, and receiving compliments on my chic but cheap outfit. I was feeling confident for a change. Jerry, usually lively, seemed uninterested in socializing and found a table near the stage. We sat and sipped merlot from plastic glasses as dentist-office-smooth jazz trailed from the ensemble on stage. I wanted to mingle, walk, dance, move—anything but sit there. I got up five or six times to fetch a bottle of water or go to the bathroom. Jerry was apparently in a mellow mood, content to sit quietly, simply listening to the music all evening. Except when he jokingly ordered me to get him another bottle of water or said, for the third time that night, "It's getting late. Isn't it past your bedtime?"

What was up with him? Was he miffed that I was out gallivanting and not sitting with him all night? Did he feel underdressed? It was only our second date. I didn't ask. What a dud he had turned out to be. But I was in too good a mood to let his sullenness get me down.

On my final return from the ladies' room, I stood outside the hospitality tent near our table, swaying to the canned commercial beat of The Manhattan Transfer, enjoying the breeze fanning in from the bay. I turned to my left to see a man next to me, smiling. Young. Gorgeous. I struck up a conversation with Mike, who told me he was from Kettering, Ohio, where I was raised. I threw out a few family names to see if he recognized anyone I grew up with, but he looked stumped. He was turning thirty-four in two weeks. No wonder. We were fifteen years apart.

As I stood talking to and enjoying Mike, our energy—the flirting so natural—I turned to glance at Jerry sitting there looking old, as if he were in Never Never Land. The last band stopped playing. It was 11:00 p.m. and Mike's friends appeared ready to leave. Jerry was still at the table alone.

"I better go be with my date," I said. "Maybe we'll see each other around on the beach."

"I hope so," he said. "Sure you can't join us after you take Grandpa home?"

Oh my God. You are so handsome. Wow! I felt a sizzle that I hadn't experienced in years. Suddenly, I had a glimpse into a more expansive world of men and dating than the one I had limited myself to. If Mike was flirting with me, I thought, perhaps other young and hot men saw me in this light, too. A big bolt of confidence shot through me, and I smiled at him as I said, "Not tonight, but maybe another time."

I walked over to the table to see if Jerry was ready to leave. He stood up and put his arm around me.

"Let's go watch the fireworks," he said.

· ✺ ·

Like clockwork, one month into a relationship I was hooked. Regardless of the roadblocks. Despite the warnings I gave myself. It was no different with Jerry. During our first four weeks of dating, he and I roller-skated the asphalt paths snaking through the county parks, walked the beaches, and took in a photography exhibit or two. Rather than dwelling on how rudely he had behaved at the Jazz Fest, I fixated instead on how wonderful it was to slow down, enjoy getting to know someone new, sit on a park bench, relax under the old live oaks, and talk about Deepak Chopra, Marianne Williamson, and the passersby. And even though I had told myself that Jerry was too old for me, when I looked at him in his Ray-Bans, his long legs stretching out from the park bench, sun streaming across his tanned face, age was no longer an issue. He was handsome, and I was feeling connected, closer to him. We were moving from the sarcastic, kidding, buddy stuff to something more meaningful.

One chilly and windy Saturday morning, the day before Halloween, it was too windy to have Yoga on the Beach. The regular instructor, Tom, was on vacation, and his substitute didn't have the key for our backup yoga studio, the church across the street. Several of us stood around trying to figure out an alternative place for an impromptu yoga class. We decided on a park down the street. I waited around to direct others to the park and then got in my car to head over there. On my way out, I saw Jerry's car pull in. I motioned him over to tell him the change in yoga plans. "Let's go get some coffee," he said.

We drove two miles down Gulf Boulevard to Lighthouse Donuts, an old-fashioned doughnut shop popular with locals and tourists alike. I grabbed one of the tables while Jerry stood in the long line to order. With a giant sugar-coated apple fritter in his left hand and a steaming cup of coffee in his right, Jerry sat down across from me and smiled.

A few days earlier I'd told him he was too defensive, so I guess he decided now was a good time to have this conversation and set the record straight. "Remember the other day when you said I was too defensive?" he said. "Well, right back at you, baby. Your armor is working overtime, trying to cover up all those wounds. We're soul mirrors. Can't you see that?"

He had mentioned the same thing at dinner a few weeks earlier.

"We're twins," he said. "We reveal each other's shadow sides." I sipped my cinnamon latte, expressionless.

Yes, I knew that all relationships help us grow and learn. From John and Patrick to Doug and Chris and the others in between, I had been fortunate to have many teachers assist me in advancing spiritually. Sometimes the clashes and power plays were obvious. Jerry pushed my buttons, as I did his. He was pumped up, prepared to have a spiritual heart-to-heart in Lighthouse Donuts. I was exhausted and wanted to sit there peacefully and not do analytics.

"I have a lot of mirrors," I said.

I don't remember exactly what I said. I know I didn't disagree with him. He was probably right. But I didn't want him to know that. He was certain enough about too many things. But I was secretly delighted knowing that he felt we had an intimate soul connection. I bet he didn't feel the same with the other women he was dating and never talked about. I suddenly felt more confident.

We'd been seeing each other for almost two months, but communications and plans with Jerry were still unpredictable. It was hard to pin him down to schedule our next get-together. When I didn't hear from him for a few days, I felt dejected, the familiar edge of abandonment creeping in. But with Jerry I didn't spend all day obsessing. I simply did what I always did: hatch a plan, lure the man to my nest with a fetching e-mail or call.

I invited him to my place on a Thursday afternoon for a walk on the beach. The evening unfolded just as the script outlined: After the walk, we came back to my house, with candles glowing, the tables adorned with glass vases of lush palm fronds, bottles of red wine opened, artisanal cheeses and sweet grapes and apples arranged just so. He reached out for me while I was slicing apples and pulled me toward him with a kiss, a meaningful, certain, passionate kiss. As Michael Bublé's seductive voice crooned in the background, Jerry pressed his body into mine hungrily, planting my back firmly against the wall, and I reached for his muscular, tanned shoulders.

"Let's go to bed," he said. "I want to make love to you." He held me and gave me a look he was sure would make me cave to his charms.

"I'm not ready yet," I said.

I wasn't going to bend. Not a chance I was going to bed with Jerry. I knew he was seeking casual sex, and I was not interested in that. Even though he was a flirt and I was aware that he had other dates, I again unknowingly created an alternative reality. The same one I always did. The one that convinced me that I was the only one he was seeing, the only one he really cared for.

"I'm getting too aroused," he said. "I have to leave."

The following week, on an early-December night, we were outside on my backyard deck entwined on the cushioned lounge chair, flames from the outdoor fireplace crackling, sipping Amaretto, when he let on about a crush he had on yet another "Unity girl." It was the first time since we'd met that I had heard him being so blatant about other women. Days later, when we ran into Yoga Tom and his wife, Tania, on the beach, I went into the bathroom to freshen up and overheard Jerry telling Tom that he had been to a singles dance the night before and it was like being a kid in a candy store, with so many pretty women to choose from.

Rather than cut it off with Jerry right then and there, I compromised, telling myself to pull back. Pull way back on my romanticism, idealism, all of those images of togetherness I had conjured. I kept thinking I could control my emotions: *I will not—do you hear me, Shary?—will not play with him anymore. I will keep it light and aloof, perhaps plan something down the road, definitely not a date. No more Amaretto and wine parties. No more fireside groping sessions. Maybe meet up for an occasional skating or yoga get-together. Probably not even that. I'm done with him.*

How naive. I needed to do more than simply will myself to change. I still did not fully grasp that to control and temper my dependency on and hunger for a man's attention and love, I had to find a substitute. I had to find other ways, healthier ways to feel good about myself.

Yet I had evolved enough to see that this runaway train Jerry and I were on was only going to lead to more and more frustration and anger. So I finally stood up for myself and stopped three months' worth of flirting, roller-skating, and fireside make-out sessions in their tracks. Four days before Christmas, it finally sank in that Jerry was behaving like a horny spring-breaker, fancying many women simultaneously.

Then it got even uglier, when I found out that he'd been out dancing every Friday night with the same woman for the past year. He had recently broken an engagement with a woman I knew nothing about. And he'd been hitting on a vulnerable, recently divorced woman in our yoga class.

I wasn't used to obeying my instincts, but with Jerry I had the courage to. Within six seconds of first seeing him that August day in the Yoga on the Beach parking lot, I told myself, *he's a player. Desperate.* And I'd been right all along. I repeatedly made promises to myself, rules about what type of man I'd get involved with and not get involved with, but they always got overridden. I went headstrong right into it with Jerry, despite my best intentions. What a losing proposition. I didn't pretend that it was anything else. I didn't want a relationship with him, but I got into one. It was the same as saying, "I don't want that drink" and then ending up having one—several—anyway. Addictions. They are all the same. We pretend we are in control. We insist we are in control.

It also became more obvious that with Jerry, like all the others, I unconsciously cancelled out my highest desires. I was in the exact same hole. Again. Lead-footed in a stew of conflicting intentions. I envisioned and prayed for a glorious, highly evolved, and powerful spiritual partner while I sloughed around the troughs in the minor leagues, this time with a man as needy, as lustful, and as addicted as I was. It wasn't satisfying anymore. I had used Jerry so I could feel desired, adored. I didn't feel good about myself anymore. It wasn't the right thing to do anymore. I'd played enough. I'd teased enough. I'd obsessed enough. I'd been intoxicated with the newness of new love possibilities. Enough.

Thankfully, I hadn't made much of an emotional investment with Jerry, nor he with me, so breaking up with him was easier—the easiest yet, in fact. My heart was bullet-holed with a legion of breakups that had walloped me to my knees with grief and depression. Was all that now a remnant of my past? True enough, I was able to let go more quickly as I had continued to reclaim rather than hand over my power. I was developing a far healthier circle of support—God, my spirit, family, and friends. With each relationship, each man, gradually I was becoming less dependent on another person for love and was cherishing and nourishing myself more. The intense relationship struggles, anguish, and drama that had propelled me through my twenties, thirties, and forties were losing their power in me. At long last, I was valuing myself and my inner peace more.

The brief interlude with Jerry represented a departure from all the other relationships: I wasn't obsessed with him. I didn't caretake or try to fix him. But what I did do was plummet to a new low: I didn't respect him. He didn't respect me. Which meant I didn't respect myself. Everything I blasted Jerry for in my journal weeks after we broke up—he's low, a snake, a common, ordinary, selfish, sleazy guy who is out to make himself feel better, fill his ego at every turn, seeking to satisfy his own desires above all else, hungry for attention, desperate to feel important, valued—was precisely the way I had operated in all my relationships. Two users seeking a fix. Jerry had been right all along. We *were* twins.

Epilogue

When did it finally dawn on me that I was addicted to love? It didn't dawn. I didn't have an epiphany. It was a slow and gradual awakening. Jerry happened to be the last straw. I was a man junkie. A relationship junkie. A romance junkie.

I went cold turkey in 2007. Dating detox. After the fling with Jerry, I vowed never to get involved with another man I didn't truly love. And I haven't been in a relationship since. I had to be *out* of a relationship to learn how to be *in* one.

And learning is what I've continued to do for the last eight years. Excavating ever deeper into my dark caves—my psyche, patterns, and history—while forging a deeper bond with God. Most essential, I'm learning to refocus the caretaking, fixing, and loving attention on myself. I loved too much all my life—in all the wrong ways, for all the wrong reasons. It's ironic, isn't it, that love addiction is not about love at all? A love addict like me unconsciously avoids love—runs like hell from healthy, real love.

I'm on the wagon, in a dry spell, a moratorium. I haven't had sex in nine years. I've not been in a relationship for eight years. I'm actually proud of my celibacy. In the past, it would have horrified me to go nine years without sex. My God! What's wrong with me? What would people think? Am I *that* unappealing? Undesirable? It used to be that to have a man look at me, want me, need me was *everything* I wanted, the only thing I needed. I hungered so much for a man's attention, touch, affirmation, and lust. It is what sustained me, made me feel alive, of value, a woman. Back then, when I wasn't in a relationship, I was as good as dead.

· ☙ ·

In the twenty-four years since my divorce, I've been on an odyssey to surface and heal my love-starved self. Like an archaeologist, I've dug inward to my truth. I have read more than a hundred self-help books. I've consulted doctors, therapists, psychics, angel readers, tarot readers, coaches, and spiritual healers. I've sung in churches, chanted with monks, meditated in temples, practiced yoga and meditation, had my soul recovered by a shaman, prayed, pleaded, journaled like a fiend, and gobbled the words of spiritual gurus as if they were my closest friends.

Almost four years ago, just playing around, I Googled "love addiction" and discovered there actually is a disorder with that name. We all hear about sex addiction. But love addiction?

According to LoveAddictionHelp.com, "By definition, an addiction or dependence is a recurring compulsion by an individual to engage in some specific behavior or activity, despite harmful consequences to the individual's health, mental state, or social life. People fall into many categories of addictions (alcohol, drugs, sex, gambling, etc.). Love addiction is one of the categories—and is a big one!"

I was flabbergasted. I found Love Addicts Anonymous (LAA) and immediately downloaded materials from the web site, particularly "Forty Questions to Help You Determine If You Are a Love Addict." According to LAA, "If you can answer yes to more than a few of the following questions, you are probably a love addict."

I responded yes to thirty-five of the forty questions. I had found my tribe.

I did not attend LAA meetings or rigidly adhere to the group's twelve steps to recovery. I did it my way. Blessedly, I had already been walking the healing path—crawling really—before I ever knew there was a twelve-step path. My way was the only way I knew. Like a sea turtle hatchling fearfully leaving its nest for the first time, scooting madly toward the water. A sea he's never swam. It's all by instinct. Just move toward the light. That's all I've done. One relationship at a time.

What have I learned?

1. What I had to learn the hard way is that love addiction is not about love at all. I thought I was being loving. I was convinced I

was. But love addiction is love avoidance according to Love Addicts Anonymous. "When you are not loving and valuing yourself, you do not have love to share with your partner. You are constantly trying to *get* love rather than share love."

2. "I am responsible for taking care of my own needs and nurturing and loving myself versus depending upon others to convince me that I'm lovable." That's from Susan Peabody's *Addiction to Love*. I am no longer searching for a relationship to give me self-worth. I've delegated that responsibility to me. Not so long ago, it occurred to me: *How in the world could I find true love when I don't have an inkling how to love?*

First I had to understand, to see that I did not love myself. I thought I did—until people close to me repeatedly pointed out ways in which I was unloving to myself. It took many relationships and many years for me to see how crucial self-love is. I thought self-love was a nice thing to have, not essential. I didn't assign it much importance. I likely had resistance to the whole idea of self-love. It was counter to the message I grew up with as an obedient Catholic girl in the 1960s: love others, be selfless, to be happy you must deny yourself. Anything else was considered selfish, a sin. I idolized the saints for their selfless acts. No one *ever* talked about self-esteem, loving, taking care of yourself back then. I also had to get, understand, what self-love meant. What is self-love really? What does it look like, sound like? When someone loves herself, how does she behave? Getting the answer took me years. I'm still trying to figure it out. Understanding that treating myself to manicures and spa trips with my mom and sisters was only scratching the surface. Over time I became aware of how much my psyche was cemented in negative, critical, diminishing, self-sabotaging thoughts and beliefs. I didn't nourish or nurture myself with kindness. Everyone else, yes. Not myself. I was gentle with others, hard on myself. Learning to be my most nurturing, kind, gentle, forgiving, understanding, encouraging, patient, and loving mother to myself was a huge learning process and everyday practice. A lifetime's worth of reprogramming is still under way.

As I moved from superficial to permanent ways of loving myself, slowly, gradually, I could—can—feel my heart expand. Enlightened ones talk about your heart opening and expanding, but I had no idea what that meant or felt like. For me, it's been an oozing of softness, a growing tenderness that's emerging. My pointy edges of self-judgment, criticism, unforgivingness—all of those hard, sharp defensive edges, like fangs and claws—are eroding.

3. I am good enough, attractive enough, important enough just as I am. I do not have to fix, help, or caretake others to earn their love.

4. When I am alone, I do not feel lonely. I am no longer afraid of being single. I love spending time alone. I am now comfortable in solitude. In fact, I crave it. For most of my life, I hated being alone and felt empty and purposeless without a man. Today I am whole, flourishing in my career, friendships, spiritual life, and creative pursuits, all of which were kicked to the curb when I was consumed with the man of the moment.

Since Jerry, I've gone out with Bruce, Mark, Fred, Jim, Patrick, Allan, and Robert—two dates each. That's it. With a few blind dates sprinkled in. My standards are higher now, and I'm better able to hold and honor my standards. Am I too picky? Yes. With dogged determination, my lifelong addiction to love has dissipated. My twelve steps have taken twenty-five years and counting.

But I know this for sure: I am a much better me. If a relationship is to be—the sacred partnership I still hope for—I am readier to love, to give love and receive love, in a far healthier and more balanced way. At fifty-seven, I'm at peace. I realize that I may never find and have the kind of partner I dream of or be the kind of partner I want to be. And I'm okay with that. I do not *need* a man. That was an impossible thought when I married John thirty years ago. It was unimaginable even seven years ago. I finally understand why lasting love has eluded me: the relationship I've been searching for all along was with myself.

Acknowledgments

I have been divinely blessed in every step of birthing this book. I am so grateful to the powerhouse She Writes Press team—Brooke Warner and Cait Levin—who shepherded me and my inaugural book with tremendous enthusiasm and care.

I would be nowhere without phenomenal teachers—wise coaches, mentors, authors and editors— by my side for the past six years. Thank you dear writing senseis:

The beautiful spirit, Bella Mahaya Carter, was my first writing coach in 2008. Bella provided a nest of encouragement, confidence and freedom for me to write what wanted to be written. With her gentle, loving support, the seed for this book was sown.

Along the way, Norma Watkins inspired me with her exquisite essays.

Jennifer Lauck first exposed me to the importance of a memoir's structure, writing as an art form and being disciplined and dedicated to the craft.

Within thirty seconds of hearing Brooke Warner speak about memoir writing on a National Association of Memoir Writers conference call in May 2012, instantly I knew I had to work with her. Brooke is the most generous, prolific, hard-working and connected coach, editor and publisher in the business. With Brooke's navigation, I was finally able to see how to transform thousands of scattered journal pages to a crisp outline to a finished manuscript. I am forever grateful.

Annie Tucker, you are a writer's dream. Every moment editing this book with you was a blast. I can't wait to collaborate with you on the next one.

Thank you, Jeff Kleiman. In our two-minute agent pitch session at the San Miguel Writers' Conference in early 2014 your feedback gave me the impetus to go back to the manuscript and whip it into something far better than what you glimpsed.

Along the way, angels appeared. One of them is lovely and selfless author advocate and agent April Eberhardt who steered me simply out of the goodness of her open heart.

My 25-year healing odyssey has been paved with an endless bounty of celestial authors, healers, therapists, counselors and shamans. Thank you for showing me the way:

A most spacious debt of appreciation to my long-time master coach and advisor, the honorable Meryl Moritz, who pulled me down from the ledge of crazy many a time. Thank you for your supreme gracefulness.

My nose was pinned to the pages of stacks of books as I searched for solace and comfort and understanding of why my love life seemed to be so cluttered with failure and unhappiness. Most profound for me have been Marianne Williamson's *Return to Love*, Wayne Dyer's *Power of Intention*, Harville Hendrix's *Receiving Love*, Deepak Chopra's *Seven Laws of Spiritual Success* and Tara Brach's *Radical Acceptance.*

Thank you to the extraordinary community of authors and healers in the love addiction community especially Robin Norwood, the author of *Women Who Love Too Much,* the first book that eloquently captured the life story of millions of readers like me. I turned to the work of Pia Mellody, Jim Hall and Brenda Schaefer frequently to understand love addiction. I am especially grateful to Susan Peabody for her immense contributions, including founding Love Addicts Anonymous (LAA), dedicating her life to writing *Addiction to Love* and counseling countless love addicts. Thank you, Susan, for your Mother Teresa-like support and encouragement.

For a brand new author, receiving advance praise from such esteemed authors as Sue William Silverman, Kerry Cohen and Ethlie Ann Vare, was manna from heaven. Thank you, dear sisters.

We all have people and circumstances throughout our lives that prompt awakening. My healing propellants happened to be my romantic relationships. When I entered an intimate relationship, the "buried sewage came rushing to the surface." Thank you, spiritual author Alan Cohen, for that visual. It fits. Thank you dear Roto-Rooters: first John, my ex-husband; then Patrick, Doug, Byron, James, Chris, and Jerry. My fundamental shape-shifters. They generated the intense and immense hurricanes that swept me under, threw me around like a nasty riptide, and spat me out, exhausted, saddened, but wiser—and so grateful for the lessons. Each time, like a Girl Scout with a new badge, I proceeded more confidently, a little less defensive and fearful, a little more open to real intimacy.

Thank you dear friends for cheering me on even when you knew very little about the particulars of this book. I am especially grateful for the most loyal and ardent Mary, Bobbi, Tania, Corinne, Ann, Rita, John, Kate, Sheila, Beth, Cathy, Coni and Rebecca. And, to Kathy, my dearest angel friend who ministered to me through most of my heart-breaks, I will always hope.

For my real-life sisters, Nancy and Patsy, I love you dearly. Thank you for standing by my side from the start of this process and sending me perpetual waves of encouragement and reassurance. Your first reads of the manuscript and initial cover designs elevated me when I needed it most.

For my beloved mother and father, Norma and Jerry Hauer, whose endless praise and love fill my now full heart. I am so incredibly blessed that I get to keep saying and sharing how much I love you. Thank you for giving me this magnificent life.

To my mother without whom this book would not be, I am grateful for your astounding wisdom which I largely dismissed most of my life. Thankfully, I finally heeded your loving urgings, "You need to write." This book is for you dear Momma.

Above all, God, who heard me sobbing 25 years ago when I was inconsolable, reeling from the devastation of being abandoned by my husband. When the only solace I could find was journaling through a torrent of tears, thrashing my anger, pain and hopelessness across the page, I wrote "Please God, let there somehow, someway be a purpose for this endless torture." Now I know the purpose was, in part, this book in your hands. Thank you for allowing me to serve You, Dear God, and those who may find meaning in these words. Namaste'.

About the Author

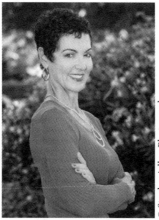

S hary Hauer is a Master Certified Executive Coach (MCC) with twenty years of success in Leadership and Executive Development with Fortune 500/1000 leaders, and the founder of The Hauer Group, a strategic consulting and coaching firm. Her business writings have been published in outlets including *Working Woman* and *HOW* magazines and *The CEO Refresher*; her creative nonfiction work has been published in *Chicken Soup for the Recovering Soul* and *Sage Woman* magazine. She lives in Clearwater Beach, Florida where she glories in the wonders of the sea, fosters feral cats, and volunteers for the hungry, homeless, and elderly. To learn more about love addiction and to connect with Shary go to: sharyhauer.com

SELECTED TITLES FROM SHE WRITES PRESS

She Writes Press is an independent publishing company
founded to serve women writers everywhere.
Visit us at www.shewritespress.com.

Where Have I Been All My Life? A Journey Toward Love and Wholeness
by Cheryl Rice $16.95, 978-1-63152-917-7
Rice's universally relatable story of how her mother's sudden death
launched her on a journey into the deepest parts of grief—and, ultimately,
toward love and wholeness.

Fire Season: A Memoir by Hollye Dexter
$16.95, 978-1-63152-974-0
After she loses everything in a fire, Hollye Dexter's life spirals downward
and she begins to unravel—but when she finds herself at the brink of
losing her husband, she is forced to dig within herself for the strength to
keep her family together.

A Leg to Stand On: An Amputee's Walk into Motherhood by Colleen Haggerty
$16.95, 978-1-63152-923-8
Haggerty's candid story of how she overcame the pain of losing a leg at
seventeen—and of terminating two pregnancies as a young woman—and
went on to become a mother, despite her fears.

Seeing Red: A Woman's Quest for Truth, Power, and the Sacred by Lone Morch
$16.95, 978-1-938314-12-4
One woman's journey over inner and outer mountains—a quest that takes
her to the holy Mt. Kailas in Tibet, through a seven-year marriage, and
into the arms of the fierce goddess Kali, where she discovers her powerful,
feminine self.

Loveyoubye: Holding Fast, Letting Go, And Then There's The Dog
by Rossandra White $16.95, 978-1-938314-50-6
A soul-searching memoir detailing the painful, but ultimately liberating,
disintegration of a twenty-five-year marriage.

Splitting the Difference: A Heart-Shaped Memoir by Tré Miller-Rodríguez
$19.95, 978-1-938314-20-9
When 34-year-old Tré Miller-Rodríguez's husband dies suddenly from
a heart attack, her grief sends her on an unexpected journey that culmi-
nates in a reunion with the biological daughter she gave up at 18.